WORKBOOK TO ACCOMPANY

HOMEMAKER/ HOME HEALTH AIDE

6th Edition

Audree Spatz
Suzann Balduzzi

Revised By
Karen O'Hara RN, BSN

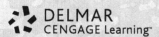
DELMAR
CENGAGE Learning™

Australia • Brazil • Japan • Korea • Mexico • Singapore • Spain • United Kingdom • United States

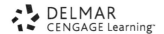

Workbook to Accompany: Homemaker/ Home Health Aide, Sixth Edition
Audree Spatz, Suzann Balduzzi
Revised by Karen O'Hara

Vice President, Health Care Business Unit:
   William Brottmiller

Editorial Director: Cathy L. Esperti

Acquisitions Editor: Marah Bellegarde

Developmental Editor: Debra Flis

Editorial Assistant: Erin Adams

Marketing Director: Jennifer McAvey

Marketing Channel Manager: Tamara Caruso

Marketing Coordinator: Kim Duffy

Project Editor: Natalie Wager

Senior Art/Design Specialist: Jay Purcell

Production Coordinator: Kenneth McGrath

ISBN-13: 978-1-4018-3142-4

ISBN-10: 1-4018-3142-7

Delmar
Executive Woods
5 Maxwell Drive
Clifton Park, NY 12065
USA

Cengage Learning is a leading provider of customized learning solutions with office locations around the globe, including Singapore, the United Kingdom, Australia, Mexico, Brazil, and Japan. Locate your local office at **www.cengage.com/global**

Cengage Learning products are represented in Canada by Nelson Education, Ltd.

To learn more about Delmar, visit **www.cengage.com/delmar**

Purchase any of our products at your local bookstore or at our preferred online store **www.cengagebrain.com**

Notice to the Reader

Printed in the United States of America
5 6 7 15 14 13 12 11

Contents

Introduction to the Learner

This workbook was written to assist you in your studies to become part of the home care team as a home health aide. Each chapter of the workbook is correlated to a unit in *Homemaker/ Home Health Aide,* Sixth Edition, and includes the following features:

- Learning Objectives remind you of important concepts learned in the text
- Terms to Define emphasize the essential terms you should be familiar with in each unit
- Application Exercises reinforce your knowledge through a variety of question-types related to the chapter content. Communication and documentation exercises and practice situations provide you with practice applying concepts learned in the text.
- Crossword puzzles give you practice learning important vocabulary.
- Chapter quizzes allow you to test your knowledge of the material in each unit.

As you develop your skills and knowledge to become a member of the health care team, you will be working under a supervisor. This supervisor could be a nurse, case manager, or other health care team member. The term *supervisor* is meant to include your direct supervisor, the person to whom you report and are supervised by. Where the term *case manager* appears, the registered nurse in charge of the client is the person being referred to.

SECTION 1

Becoming a Home Health Aide

UNIT 1   HOME HEALTH SERVICES

LEARNING OBJECTIVES

After studying this unit, you should be able to:
- Name four reasons why the need for home care is increasing
- Discuss the role of a home health aide
- List five nursing procedures provided by the home health aide
- Name members and functions of various members of the home care team
- Name four health care workplaces outside of the hospital setting
- Give an example of a managed care organization
- List four different types of illnesses or disabilities a client might have
- List three programs that assist in paying for health care costs
- List two requirements of the Omnibus Budget Reconciliation Act (OBRA) that affect you as a home health aide

TERMS TO DEFINE

- acute illness
- adult day-care center
- assisted living center
- Background Information Disclosure Form
- case manager (CM)
- chronic illness
- companion
- culture
- developmentally disabled
- diagnosis-related group (DRG)
- diversity
- enterostomal therapist (RN, ET)
- health care provider
- hospice
- licensed practical nurse (LPN)
- long-term care facility

- long-term care insurance
- managed care
- Medicaid
- Medicare
- Nurse Aide Registry
- nurse practitioner (NP)
- occupational therapist (OT)
- Omnibus Budget Reconciliation Act (OBRA)
- Outcome and Assessment Information Set (OASIS)
- personal care worker
- physical therapist (PT)
- Prospective Payment System (PPS)
- registered dietitian (RD)
- registered nurse (RN)
- respiratory therapist (RRT)

■ respite care
■ social worker (BSW, MSW)

■ speech therapist (ST)
■ terminal illness

APPLICATION EXERCISES

Short Answer/Fill in the Blanks. *Complete the following sentences with the correct word or words.*

1. The main purpose of the first homemaker service agency in the United States was to provide _____ _____.

2. Home health aides are expected to work under direct supervision of a _____ _____.

3. Minimum training and competency requirements for home health aides were established by the _____ _____ _____ _____, also known as _____.

4. In the earlier years of our country the elderly and people with disabilities were cared for by _____ members.

5. As the country became industrialized, the family unit became smaller, usually consisting of the parents and the children only. This type of family is known as the _____ family.

6. One of the main reasons for the growth of home care is the growth in the _____ _____, the main recipients of home care.

7. Once an individual completes the home health aide training program and passes the competency test, he or she is placed on the _____ _____ _____ _____ in which they reside.

8. Many people prefer to remain in their own _____ rather than move to a _____ _____ when they become ill or frail.

9. Home care services for people who prefer to remain at home to die are called _____.

10. Two main categories of duties of home care workers are care of the _____ and care of the _____.

11. Activities of daily living include:
    a. _____
    b. _____
    c. _____
    d. _____

12. Care of the home environment can include:
    a. _____
    b. _____
    c. _____
    d. _____

13. Each home care client has a separate care plan that is designed by the worker's _____ _____.

14. The home health aide is a member of the health care _____.

15. A federally and state funded program that pays for health care services for persons whose income is below a certain amount is _____.

16. To qualify for Medicare reimbursement for home health care, an individual must be:

   a. confined to _____.

   b. under the care of a _____.

   c. in need of _____ _____ _____,
      _____ _____, or _____
      _____.

   d. receiving care from a Medicare _____ _____.

17. Everyone in the United States who has paid into _____ _____ is entitled to apply for Medicare insurance if they were born before _____ or become _____.

18. The method of health care delivery that attempts to control costs through the use of gatekeepers controlling access to care is called a _____ _____ _____. They are sometimes referred to as _____ _____.

19. It is crucial that the _____ _____ _____ report and document any change in the condition of each individual client in order for the patient to have quality care and the agency to receive adequate reimbursement.

Matching. *Match each term with the correct definition.*

20. ____ companion

21. ____ home care aide

22. ____ home health aide

23. ____ personal care worker

24. ____ homemaker/home health aide

25. ____ homemaker

a. assists in general household tasks, as well as those listed for the home health aide

b. performs household duties such as laundry and cooking

c. works with the client with the goal of assisting the client with independent living under professional supervision

d. keeps the client company or helps to maintain safety, usually does not provide personal or homemaking services

e. assists with a minimal level of daily living activities, such as meal preparation and companionship as well as minimal assistance with personal care

f. able to provide substantial assistance with personal care, such as bathing and dressing

True or False. *Answer the following statements true (T) or false (F).*

26. T F The Omnibus Reconciliation Act (OBRA) mandates federal Medicare and Medicaid standards for nursing homes and home health care agencies.

27. T F A mutual goal of the OBRA, Medicare, and Medicaid regulations is to improve care for individuals in long-term care facilities and for those in their homes.

28. T F Medicare is a state program.

29. T F The physical therapist authorizes home health care.

30. T F Home health care clients are diverse and represent many different cultures and ethnic groups.

31. T F A chronic illness is one that lasts a short time, requires immediate treatment, and can be expected to go away.

32. T F Alzheimer's disease is considered a chronic illness.

33. T F Developmentally disabled means a severe chronic disability developing before age 21.

34. T F Terminal illnesses are illnesses that individuals are expected to recover from in a short time.

35. T F Home health care clients come from all ages, all cultures, and all ethnic groups.

36. T F Home health aides must be willing to listen to the instructions from their case managers regarding the care of each individual because they cannot expect to know all the different traditions and practices of each client.

37. T F A home health aide must instruct the client to follow the religious practices of the home health aide.

38. T F A speech therapist assesses the client's ability to stand, walk, and climb stairs.

39. T F An occupational therapist evaluates a client's ability to perform activities of daily living.

40. T F A social worker gives direct nursing care to the client.

Multiple Choice. *Choose the correct answer or answers.*

41. Increased need for home care is due to
   a. the increase of HMOs
   b. the shortage of hospital beds
   c. discharge of clients that are sicker and need follow-up care
   d. the shortage of health care providers

42. The person who evaluates the client's ability to perform skills necessary to independent living is the
   a. physical therapist
   b. occupational therapist
   c. speech therapist
   d. home health aide

43. A federally and state-funded program that pays for health care services for those persons with income below a certain level is called
   a. Medicaid
   b. Medicare
   c. HMOs
   d. food stamps

44. Whenever government funding is involved in health care
    a. there will be much waste
    b. federal regulation of the health care industry will be present
    c. the states will not be involved in regulation
    d. each state will determine its own requirements
45. The person responsible for coordinating the care of the client is
    a. the home health aide   c. the case manager
    b. the social worker   d. the office supervisor

PRACTICE SITUATIONS

Case 1

Joan, a friend of yours, approaches you and tells you she is going to have surgery in the next few weeks. Her health care provider has told her that she will need help after going home. She knows you are becoming a home health aide. She asks you to explain what you do in the home for your clients. She is nervous about having strangers in her home.

Questions

1. What information can you give Joan to make her feel more comfortable about care in the home?
2. Do home health care agencies have to be licensed?
3. Who are the members of the home health care team?

Case 2

You have worked for 10 years in a nursing home as a certified nurse's assistant. Your employer goes out of business. Someone tells you about a home health care agency that is hiring staff.

Questions

1. What would you do to find out more about home health care?
2. What certification would you need?
3. Name five home health aide functions you may be asked to demonstrate to an employer.

CROSSWORD PUZZLE

Across

1 member of the health care team who coordinates all the services the client may require

4 performs personal and nursing care skills

6 health care worker that keeps the client company, no hands-on care

8 the learned behavior patterns of a race, nation, or people

12 assesses the client's condition and determines the type of personal and nursing care needed; provides care

Down

2 assesses the client's ability to communicate, understand, and write; works to rehabilitate the client

3 illness that lasts a long time

5 insurance that pays for medical care for clients over age 65 and disabled

7 begins suddenly and is usually severe

9 group that cares for dying clients and their families

10 final life-ending stage

11 Omnibus Budget Reconciliation Act

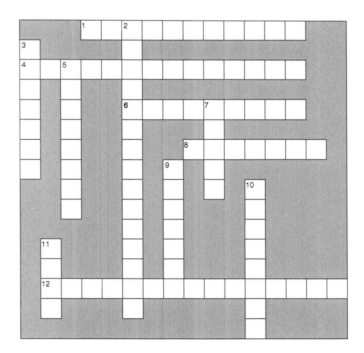

UNIT QUIZ

True or False. *Answer the following statements true (T) or false (F).*

1. T   F   Acute illness comes on suddenly and has a short duration.
2. T   F   Many individuals with disabilities will be able to tell you what you need to do for them.
3. T   F   It is okay to do everything for clients while you are there because it would take forever to let them do it for themselves.
4. T   F   People with physical disabilities may display periods of hopelessness.
5. T   F   It is important for you as a homemaker/home health aide to present a positive attitude toward the client and the family.
6. T   F   The Prospective Payment System established minimum training and competency requirements for home health aides.
7. T   F   Respiratory therapists assist clients with any breathing problems.
8. T   F   A dietician provides instruction in speech exercises and swallowing.
9. T   F   Bereavement counseling is an important part of hospice care.
10. T   F   An enterostomal therapist (RN, ET) is a specialist who works with clients who have ostomies or clients who require special skin care.

Short Answer/Fill in the Blanks. *Complete the following sentences with the correct word or words.*

11. A _____ or _____ is a nurse who is licensed by the state to practice nursing.
12. A _____ _____, like cerebral palsy is an example of a long-term health problem.
13. A residential home for individuals who need twenty-four-hour skilled care is a

    _____ _____ _____ _____.

14. A _____ _____ _____ works with clients the most.
15. _____ are studies done to determine the number of days of hospitalization necessary for certain medical conditions.
16. Home health aides are expected to work under direct supervision of a _____

    _____.
17. Four health care workplaces outside of the hospital setting are _____,

    _____, _____, and _____.
18. Three programs that assist in paying for health care costs are _____,

    _____, and _____.
19. Five nursing procedures provided by the home health aide are _____,

    _____, _____, _____, and _____.
20. _____ _____ _____ can be defined as all those services that promote, maintain, and restore physical, social, or emotional health to clients in the home setting.

UNIT 2   HOME HEALTH AIDE RESPONSIBILITIES AND LEGAL RIGHTS

LEARNING OBJECTIVES

After studying this unit, you should be able to:

- List three important qualities of the home health aide
- Give five examples of actions to avoid that can lead to liability
- Give examples of good personal hygiene
- Define ethics, and identify two examples of ethical practice
- Define the following legal terms—aiding and abetting, defamation, assault, battery, and malpractice
- Describe eight "rights of clients"
- Describe eight "rights of home health aides"
- Explain the purpose of the Health Insurance Portability and Accountability Act
- Define client abuse
- List four types of client abuse and give an example of each
- Discuss what to do if you suspect client abuse

TERMS TO DEFINE

- abandonment
- abuse
- aiding and abetting
- assault
- battery
- career
- confidentiality
- defamation
- ethics
- evaluation
- false imprisonment
- flexible
- Health Insurance Portability and Accountability Act (HIPAA)
- hygiene
- interaction
- interpersonal relationships
- invasion of privacy
- involuntary seclusion
- liability
- libel
- malpractice
- negligence
- ombudsman
- procedure
- slander
- theory

APPLICATION EXERCISES

Short Answer/Fill in the Blanks. *Complete the following sentences with the correct word or words.*

1. A _____ is an occupation or profession for which one has been specially educated.

2. A home health aide must be flexible, be willing to follow instructions, be _____ organized, dependable and _____, have good _____ skills, be _____, _____, and have good personal _____.

3. A home health aide must be able to adjust _____ from one situation to another.

4. The home health aide must treat all clients with _____.

5. The home health aide must be able to _____ to different settings and be able to give _____ and _____ care in each situation.

6. An _____ may consist of written tests or demonstrations where you perform an actual procedure and are assessed if done correctly.

7. A _____ is a list of steps used to complete a task.

8. _____ is the information that forms a basis for action.

9. _____ is the actual performance of the procedure.

10. Before assigning a client, the _____ will provide a home care plan for the client, describing the specific duties of the home health aide.

11. The care plan should include duties, client's needs, and the _____ to _____ in case of an emergency.

12. _____ refers to the degree to which you will be held financially responsible for the damages resulting from your negligence.

13. Do only and exactly what your case manager _____ instructs you to do.

14. Pitfalls you should avoid in your job include:

    a. doing _____ than is assigned

    b. doing _____ than is assigned

    c. doing _____, _____, or poor quality work

    d. using your car for _____ _____ without notifying your _____ company

    e. failing to act in an _____

    f. failing to do accurate and daily reporting and _____

    g. attempting to do things that are beyond your _____

    h. _____ yourself or your client by doing something you are not assigned or adequately trained to do

    i. failing to report unsafe _____

15. A home health aide will usually be assigned to more than one client; for the aide to complete the tasks in the proper time frame, the aide will have to be _____.

16. Interactions occur between one or more _____.

17. The home health aide may be the first to notice a _____ with the client.

18. Personal appearance guidelines for the home health aide include to bathe _____, use _____, do not wear _____ perfumes or aftershave, and _____ your teeth regularly.

19. Fingernails should be _____ and _____.

20. Bracelets, _____ earrings and necklaces, and large stone rings should not be worn in the client's home because disoriented clients might grab them and a large ring can _____ a client's skin.

21. Clients with lung disease, allergies, respiratory illness, or personal distaste for the smell of cigarettes may have an _____ _____ to cigarette smoke.

22. This act was created to develop guidelines and _____ transmitting information that identified individual clients _____.

23. _____ is a code or standard of behavior. It is a code concerned with what is _____ and what is _____.

24. Dishonesty not only involves the taking of objects or money, but also means not _____ reports.

25. Home health aides should _____ discuss their clients with anyone except their supervisors.

26. If a client offers you a gift, you should do what? _____

27. If a client becomes rude, what would you do to handle it? _____

28. Medicare and Medicaid have mandated a list of rights of clients that must be given to each client that is funded by the government. Five of them are:

    a. _____

    b. _____

    c. _____

    d. _____

    e. _____

29. Eight rights you have as a home health aide are:

    a. _____

    b. _____

    c. _____

    d. _____

    e. _____

    f. _____

    g. _____

    h. _____

30. Client abuse may be:

    a. _____

    b. _____

    c. _____

    d. _____

True or False. *Answer the following statements true (T) or false (F).*

31. T   F   The home health aide is the person who spends the least amount of time with the client.

32. T   F   The client becomes confused; the client was not confused earlier. The home health aide should contact the health care provider.

33. T   F   The home where the client lives may be upset before the home health aide arrives; the home health aide should leave if it is too bad.

34. T   F   If the client asks the home health aide to take her to the store shopping, the home health aide should assist the client to the car.

35. T   F   If the client asks the home health aide to join her for lunch, the aide should politely tell the client that this is not allowed by the agency, that the aide's role is to assist the client.

36. T   F   It is always better to report something you are not sure of than to not report it.

Matching. *Match each description with the correct legal term.*

37. ____ being left without care or support by family or agency

38. ____ act of touching of a person's body without consent

39. ____ stating untrue statements about a person that would injure the person's name or reputation

40. ____ not reporting dishonest acts that one observed

41. ____ an intentional attempt or threat to touch a person without the person's consent

a. abandonment

b. aiding and abetting

c. assault

d. battery

e. defamation

Practical Exercises. *In the following list of items, mark 1 if it needs to be reported to your case manager or mark 2 if it does not need to be reported to your case manager.*

42. ____ The client fell down but was not injured.

43. ____ The telephone does not work.

44. ____ The garbage has not been taken out for a week.

45. ____ The client's daughter dropped off her 2-year-old child for you to watch.

46. ____ The client asks you to work on your day off and asks you not to tell the agency.

47. ____ You notice a large amount of blood in the toilet after the client has used it.

48. ____ The client complains that you are not the regular assistant.

49. ____ The client complains about the brand of dishwashing liquid you purchased.

50. ____ The client requests that you take him or her shopping.

51. ____ The client asks you to wash the dog.

Multiple Choice. *Choose the correct answer or answers.*

52. When caring for a client in the home, it is expected that you
    a. watch the client's favorite television shows with the client
    b. share your feelings regarding the client's concerns about other family members
    c. will use the client's telephone to take care of your necessary tasks
    d. none of these

53. If the client asks the aide to perform duties that have not been assigned by the case manager, the aide
    a. should do what the client requests
    b. can tell what needs to be done
    c. needs to contact the case manager before proceeding
    d. should refuse to perform these tasks

54. The home health aide should be properly groomed at all times. This includes
    a. clean clothing and shoes   c. polished shoes
    b. trimmed fingernails   d. all of these

55. Important instructions that the home health aide needs to know before taking care of the client include
    a. how and who to report information to
    b. how much the client is paying for the aide's services
    c. what kind of laundry detergent the client uses
    d. how the client was referred to the agency

56. If the client is unhappy with the home health aide, the aide should
    a. leave and go somewhere else
    b. tell the client that she will just have to be satisfied because the aide was assigned to her
    c. try to determine why the client is unhappy
    d. report to the case manager

PRACTICE SITUATIONS

Case 1

You are assigned to care for Mr. Lopez. When you arrive at Mr. Lopez's home, you are greeted by his daughter. She tells you that you are to make sure he takes his bath. When you enter Mr. Lopez's room to prepare for his bath, he tells you he is not taking a bath. You are aware that the client has the right to refuse care.

Questions

1. What will you do?

2. What will you tell his daughter?

3. Do you need to contact your case manager?

Case 2

While you are caring for Mr. Lopez, he urinates on the floor. He has not been incontinent before. While you are cleaning up the accident, he informs you not to tell anyone, in particular his daughter. Mr. Lopez tells you his daughter will put him in a nursing home if she finds out.

Questions

1. What is the right thing to do?
2. You are expected to inform your case manager. Can you do this without telling Mr. Lopez?
3. What about Mr. Lopez's daughter, are you obligated to tell her?

CROSSWORD PUZZLE

Across

2 standard or code of behavior

6 the reciprocating actions between two people or between members of a group

7 gathering information about changes in the client's condition or behavior; using your five senses

9 treatment that reasonably could cause physical pain, mental anguish, or fear

10 action on your part or failure to act which causes physical injury or property damage

Down

1 being left without care

3 personal cleanliness of the human body

4 to record on proper form your observations and actions

5 to make a written record or oral summary of the care of a client

7 person from the state department who investigates and mediates client problems that have been reported

8 the practical and necessary information one must learn about a subject

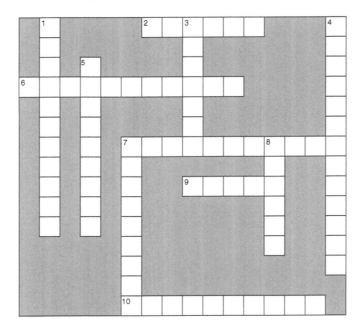

UNIT QUIZ

Multiple Choice. *Choose the correct answer or answers.*

1. If you are unsure of the correct terminology to use on the medical record, you should notify the
   a. case manager
   b. physical therapist
   c. supervisor
   d. medical social worker

2. You see that it is getting much more difficult to transfer the client into the bathtub. You should
   a. tell the daughter she must stay home from work
   b. arrange for a neighbor to help you lift the client
   c. notify your supervisor or client's case manager per agency policy
   d. call 911 for assistance

3. All of these are examples of abuse except for
   a. screaming at a client
   b. involuntary seclusion
   c. no telephone service
   d. pinching or slapping a person

4. Arriving at lunchtime, you are prioritizing your care for Mrs. Panczenka, a client with osteoarthritis who is bedbound. On arrival, she is clean and neat but complaining of being hungry. Which task should you perform first?
   a. wash the client's clothes and soiled linens
   b. prepare lunch and serve meal to client
   c. bathe client
   d. change dry dressing on client's arm

5. Circle all the situations that home health aides should avoid
   a. doing more than is assigned
   b. being punctual for work
   c. doing less than is assigned
   d. attempting to do things that are beyond your abilities

6. Guidelines for personal appearance of the home health aide include all of the following except
   a. bathe daily and use deodorant
   b. wear makeup moderately
   c. long acrylic sculpted nails are acceptable
   d. no dangling bracelets or necklaces

7. Ethical standards include all but
   a. respect the cultural and religious practices of the client and family
   b. keeping tips and gifts
   c. never walk out in the middle of an assignment
   d. keeping accurate records of client care activities and time in the home

8. Professional standards of behavior include
   a. be dependable and reliable
   b. show respect for client's privacy and modesty
   c. control any negative reactions to chronic disability or the living conditions of the client
   d. all of the above

9. Client's rights include

    a. client shall be treated with consideration, respect, and full recognition of the client's dignity and individuality

    b. client has the right to be free from mental and physical abuse

    c. client has the right to refuse treatment after being fully informed of and understanding the consequences of such action

    d. all of the above

Matching. *Match each term with the correct definition.*

10. ____ evaluation

11. ____ procedure

12. ____ practice

13. ____ theory

14. ____ assault

15. ____ negligence

16. ____ battery

17. ____ slander

18. ____ abandonment

19. ____ libel

a. false written statement about another

b. a client being left without care

c. failure to act; forgetting to do a task

d. making an oral false statement about another

e. touching a person without the person's consent

f. a list of steps to complete a task

g. actual performance of procedures

h. information that forms a basis for action

i. threat to touch a person

j. written tests or demonstration of procedure

UNIT 3 DEVELOPING EFFECTIVE COMMUNICATION SKILLS AND DOCUMENTATION

LEARNING OBJECTIVES

After studying this unit, you should be able to:

- Explain why health care team members need to communicate
- Describe guidelines for effective communication
- Explain the importance of positive feedback
- List barriers to communication
- Acquaint oneself with methods to communicate with clients from a different culture, clients who are hard-of-hearing, or clients who have limited vision
- List basic rules for charting
- Interpret medical abbreviations and vocabulary words
- Explain the meaning of the "twenty-four-hour clock"
- Explain contents of the "Client Plan of Care"
- Identify information that can be collected about a client using sight, hearing, touch, smell, and taste
- Explain how you would answer the client's phone

TERMS TO DEFINE

- active listening
- body language
- communication
- cultural diversity
- documentation
- invalidate
- listening
- nonjudgmental

- nonverbal communication
- objective
- observation
- paraphrasing
- passive listening
- platitude
- report
- subjective

APPLICATION EXERCISES

Short Answer/Fill in the Blanks. *Complete the following sentences with the correct word or words.*

1. Effective _____ may be the most important skill that a care provider can learn.

2. _____ is defined as the behaviors, values, beliefs, habits, and customs of a group of people.

3. Often the stress of _____ and _____ brings changes in the behavior of family members.

4. Communication is the successful transmission of a message from one _____ to a _____.

5. The communication process involves a message sent by the _____ and received by the _____. For communication to successfully take place, the message sent and the message received must be the _____.

6. Praising someone for doing the right thing or for doing something well is called

   _____ _____.

7. The three key aspects of communication include how messages are _____ and

   _____, _____ _____, and

   _____ _____.

8. Eye contact, body language, and gestures are examples of _____

   _____.

9. Four techniques for improving communication with clients with hearing, speech, or visual impairments are:

   a. _____

   b. _____

   c. _____

   d. _____

10. Touching someone is a method of _____ communication.

11. _____ is difficult when there are loud noises or when the receiver is distracted.

12. _____ is an excellent way to learn about the client and family.

13. Five tools of effective listening are:

   a. _____

   b. _____

   c. _____

   d. _____

   e. _____

14. Communication in the workplace is essential. The health care worker needs to be able to communicate clearly with coworkers. Three examples of information that the home health aide would need to communicate to coworkers are:

    a. _____

    b. _____

    c. _____

15. The health care worker also must communicate clearly with the client. Three examples of information that the worker needs to communicate clearly to the client are:

    a. _____

    b. _____

    c. _____

16. Four active listening behaviors that are helpful in clear communication include:

    a. _____

    b. _____

    c. _____

    d. _____

17. The _____ _____ _____ is a legal document that is constructed by the case manager, in conjunction with the client's health care provider, and implemented by the home health aide and other direct care staff.

18. List six basic rules for recording your report.

    a. _____

    b. _____

    c. _____

    d. _____

    e. _____

    f. _____

19. A client _____ needs to be reported immediately.

20. List eight abnormal signs and symptoms that need to be reported and documented.

    a. _____

    b. _____

    c. _____

    d. _____

    e. _____

    f. _____

    g. _____

    h. _____

True or False. *Answer the following statements true (T) or false (F).*

21. T F If the client is talking about a subject that the home health aide finds depressing, it is acceptable for the aide to change the subject.

22. T F Passive listening, rushing to answer the speaker before he or she is finished, and interrupting the speaker are all examples of poor listening.

23. T F The client is talking about how sad she feels because her arthritis is causing her a great deal of pain. It is appropriate for the home health aide to tell her, "Tomorrow's another day."

24. T F Yes or no questions are a good way to show the client that you are interested in the dialogue.

25. T F Asking clients to advise you on a personal matter is good because it takes their mind off themselves.

26. T F "Why" questions are a way of judging another person.

27. T F Paying close attention to the speaker is a good listening skill.

28. T F Active listening is a tool that will help the worker become involved in the communication process.

29. T F It is acceptable to assume that we know what the speaker is saying.

30. T F Paraphrasing what you heard means restating in your own words what the other person has said.

Communication Exercises. *Write the appropriate response to the following remarks.*

31. "You do not have to cook for me today; I want you to take me to the mall instead."

32. "I have a terrible feeling that something bad is going to happen."

33. "You know that Bertha down the hall, she steals everything I get from my daughter."

34. "I am going to die soon, but nobody will tell me the truth."

Abbreviation Exercises. *Next to each phrase, write the appropriate abbreviation.*

35. every three hours _____

36. twice a day _____

37. nothing by mouth _____

38. intake and output _____

39. hour of sleep _____

40. blood pressure _____

41. every other day _____

42. short of breath _____

43. immediately _____

44. when needed or necessary _____

45. bowel movement _____

46. temperature, pulse, respirations _____

47. by mouth _____

48. without _____

49. complains of _____

50. activities of daily living _____

51. wheelchair _____

52. discontinue _____

53. with _____

54. every day _____

Multiple Choice. *Choose the correct answer or answers.*

55. Many factors could affect receiving messages correctly. These include
    a. hearing loss
    b. distracting noise in the room
    c. depression
    d. all of these

56. Nonverbal communication includes
    a. the words the speaker says
    b. the look on the face of the speaker
    c. the language the speaker speaks
    d. none of these

57. If the client has hearing loss, the aide should
    a. speak clearly
    b. use short sentences
    c. write when able to
    d. all of these

58. Examples of close-ended questions include
    a. "Tomorrow's another day."
    b. "I can see you are upset by this."
    c. "Do you want to go outside?"
    d. "Why do you think your son is upset?"

59. Communication requires
    a. speaker
    b. receiver
    c. message
    d. all of these

60. An example of asking for more information is
    a. "I'm interested, tell me more."
    b. "I know that you are upset, but there is nothing I can do."
    c. "Today after we finish with your exercises, I'm going to take you for a walk."
    d. "You look cheerful today."

Matching. *Match each term with the correct definition.*

61. ____ sputum		a. scrapes
62. ____ rales		b. no appetite
63. ____ quadriplegia		c. bruises
64. ____ purulent		d. large amount
65. ____ productive		e. pressure sores/ulcer
66. ____ paraplegia		f. difficulty in breathing
67. ____ hemiplegia		g. swelling
68. ____ hematuria		h. walking style
69. ____ abrasions		i. paralysis on one side of the body
70. ____ anorexia		j. paralysis from the waist down
71. ____ contusions		k. coughing up material
72. ____ copious		l. pus-like drainage
73. ____ decubitus ulcer		m. paralysis from the neck down
74. ____ dyspnea		n. moist respiration
75. ____ edema		o. phlegm—spit
76. ____ gait		p. blood in urine

Documentation Exercises. *Read the following descriptions and provide documentation for each scenario.*

77. You arrive at your client's house and as you walk in you see your client sitting in a chair crying. You ask her what is wrong. She shrugs her shoulders and continues to cry. How would you document this?

78. You prepare lunch for your client. As he starts to eat, you notice that he is putting a large amount of salt on his food. Your case manager has instructed you that the client's food is to be served without any added salt. How would you document this?

79. You notice your client is feeling warm. You check her temperature. It is 100°F. As you look closely at her, you notice her face is flushed and she feels warm when you touch her. How would you document this?

PRACTICE SITUATIONS

Case 1

You arrive at your client's house. Mr. Long looks very sad. You ask him what is wrong. He tells you that his dog has been hit by a car and is dead. He states, "Spot was the only person left that loved me. Now I am all alone."

Questions

1. What will you say to him?
2. Can you think of anything to cheer him up?

Case 2

You are assigned to care for Mrs. Kay. She requires a bath, meal preparation, and laundry to be washed. When you arrive, her daughter is there with three children, all in diapers. She immediately starts telling you what she requires you to do. Feed her children, wash the laundry that she brought, and clean the kitchen. You know that you are being paid by Medicare to care only for your client. Mrs. Kay is frightened and cannot explain your role to her daughter.

Questions

1. How will you make sure your client is cared for and not intimidated by her daughter?
2. What will you do about all the expectations of Mrs. Kay's daughter?

When you explain to Mrs. Kay's daughter that you are being paid by Medicare to care for her mother, she informs you that all of the other home health aides do as she asks.

3. What is your ethical obligation regarding this information?

Case 3

You are assigned to care for Mrs. Peterson who is recovering from a broken hip. The client insists that you give her a tub bath, even though the plan of care states that she should have a sponge bath.

Questions

1. What should you do next?
2. What do you report to the case manager?
3. What should you document?

CROSSWORD PUZZLE

Across

1 offering reassurances that are not valid to another person

5 those changes reported by the client that are not visible

6 communicating without words using gestures, expressions, or body movement

9 restating in your own words what the other person has said

10 without placing value judgment on the actions or words of others

Down

2 listening to the speaker, reflecting the speaker's feelings, and commenting on them to the speaker

3 a form of communication using gestures and facial expressions instead of words

4 the sending and receiving of messages, may be verbal or nonverbal

7 documenting on the chart or informing the case manager of abnormal signs or symptoms

8 hearing with thoughtful attention

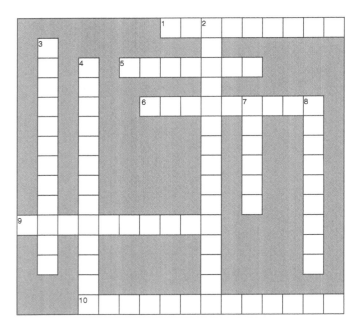

UNIT QUIZ

True or False. *Answer the following statements true (T) or false (F).*

1. T   F   Communication involves how messages are sent and received, active listening, and nonverbal communication.

2. T   F   Observation skills involving the five senses: seeing, hearing, touching, smelling, and tasting should be used in the day-to-day work of the home health aide.

3. T   F   A negative statement should come before a positive action the client is doing so the client will remember the last thing said.

4. T F Hearing loss, medications, disabilities, and depression have only minor effects on how a client receives communication.

5. T F Clients with hearing, speech, or visual impairments need special attention.

6. T F Platitudes such as "Oh, you'll get over it" may completely invalidate the client's feelings.

7. T F You do not need to report unwitnessed client falls to your case manager.

8. T F It is acceptable to document using a regular lead pencil in charting.

9. T F If you make a mistake in charting, erase it or use correction fluid to fix the mistake.

10. T F It is important to sign and date every medical record entry as a home health aide.

Matching. *Match each phrase with the correct abbreviation.*

11. _____ temperature, pulse, respiration   a. BM

12. _____ short of breath   b. pc

13. _____ when needed or necessary   c. SOB

14. _____ nothing by mouth   d. TPR

15. _____ after meals   e. prn

16. _____ intake and output   f. NPO

17. _____ bowel movement   g. I&O

Fill in the Blanks. *Complete the following sentences with the correct word or words.*

18. A _____ _____ is a pressure sore or ulcer caused by lack of movement and prolonged pressure on a body part.

19. Mrs. Edwards who has chronic obstructive pulmonary disease has _____, which is difficulty in breathing.

20. Stephen was in an auto accident, which severed his cervical spine resulting in _____, paralysis from the neck down.

21. Wheelchair-bound Mr. Santos has paraplegia, _____ _____ _____ _____ _____.

22. Clients with congestive heart failure often have _____ or swelling in the legs.

23. Mr. Montegro has liver failure causing his eyes and skin to be _____ or yellow.

24. Clients with depression may be withdrawn meaning _____ _____ _____ _____.

25. Urinary tract infections may cause clients to have _____, blood in their urine.

UNIT 4   SAFETY

LEARNING OBJECTIVES

After studying this unit, you should be able to:

- Identify the conditions in aging that contribute to the incidence of accidents
- Identify five causes of accidents around the home
- List five precautions to use when a client is receiving oxygen
- List four ways to make the home safer for a client with dementia
- Discuss the various types of fire extinguishers
- Discuss home health aide safety outside the client's home
- State the basic rules to follow in the event of a home fire
- List five safety tips for the home

TERMS TO DEFINE

- evacuate
- fire extinguisher
- emergency medical technician (EMT)
- hazard

- PASS
- peripheral vision
- RACE

APPLICATION EXERCISES

Short Answer/Fill in the Blanks. *Complete the following sentences with the correct word or words.*

1. Human factors are directly related to many home _____.

2. Home health aides should be aware of the many causes of accidents in the _____.

3. Painkillers or tranquilizers may make the client unsteady; they may need _____ ambulating.

4. If the client is taking more than one medication, sometimes the medications _____, causing disorientation or unsteady balance.

5. Clients can also become _____ and not remember whether they have taken their medication.

6. According to the National Safety Council, at least one person in _____ suffers some kind of injury as a result of an accident that takes place in someone's home.

7. As the body ages, the bones become brittle and _____ easily.

8. Five ways to make the home environment safer are:

   a. _____

   b. _____

   c. _____

   d. _____

   e. _____

9. One of the most dangerous rooms in the house is the _____.

10. Some hazards may be avoided by providing a _____ _____.

11. Many elderly clients get up at _____ to use the bathroom. It is advisable to keep a _____ on in the bathroom.

12. Older adults lose their _____ vision. This means that they can see things _____ _____ only.

13. When a client is wearing a cast, the home health aide should check around the cast frequently for signs of _____ and _____.

14. If the home health aide notices any unsafe conditions in the client's home, the aide should contact the _____ immediately.

15. All homes should be equipped with a _____ _____ in case of fire.

16. If a fire occurs, the home health aide should remember that smoke rises, and if the client cannot be safely moved, the aide should cover the client's face with a _____ _____ and try to move the client to a _____ _____ _____.

17. Smoke rises, and if it is inhaled for a long time, it can cause _____.

18. There are _____ main types of fire extinguishers.

19. If a fire extinguisher is used, it must be held _____ and the nozzle aimed at the _____ edge of the fire.

20. Once a fire extinguisher is used, it must be _____.

21. List five safety checklist items.

   a. _____

   b. _____

   c. _____

   d. _____

   e. _____

22. Homes with toddlers should have unused _____ _____ covered with plugs.

23. Medications should be stored out of the reach of _____.

24. The elderly are at-risk for burn injury due to decreased nerve impulses or _____ _____.

25. List five basic rules for the home health aide to follow in case of fire in the client's home.

    a. _____

    b. _____

    c. _____

    d. _____

    e. _____

26. List five tips to make a home safer for a client with dementia.

    a. _____

    b. _____

    c. _____

    d. _____

    e. _____

True or False. *Answer the following statements true (T) or false (F).*

27. T   F   Animals in the home are directly related to most home accidents.

28. T   F   Scatter rugs should have a nonskid backing or be removed from the home.

29. T   F   Use the word RACE to remember what to do when faced with a fire situation.

30. T   F   Friends and relatives of a client using oxygen may smoke as long as they are 20 feet away from the client.

31. T   F   Clients with dementia should have an ID bracelet containing medical information and a phone number.

32. T   F   Hot water temperature should be about 140°F to prevent burns while bathing.

33. T   F   Elderly clients with poor balance need safety rails or a shower chair in the tub.

Matching. *Match the type of accidents with the age group that they are frequently seen in.*

34. _____ injuries from auto, motorbike, or bicycle; accidents due to carelessness, drunkenness, or drug abuse; wounds from gun accidents

35. _____ falls

36. _____ burns from careless use of outside fire, and inside fireplace; from overloading electrical circuits; from smoking in bed

37. _____ falls from a table or a bedside

38. _____ scalding from pulling pot handles on stove

39. _____ injuries from bicycle and auto accidents; hit by car when darting into street

a. infants up to 1 year

b. preschool children

c. preteen children

d. teenagers

e. adults

f. old age

Documentation Exercises. *Read the following descriptions and provide documentation for each scenario.*

40. You have taken your client for a walk. She walks using a walker. After she has traveled one block, she becomes very short of breath. After a brief resting period, she is able to walk back to her home. How would you document the walk?

41. You are bathing a bedbound client and notice cigarette ashes in her bed and burn holes on her nightgown. How would you document this information? Who should you notify?

42. Arriving at Mr. Jones's home, his wife informs you, "John fell again last night transferring from his wheelchair into bed. He's not hurt." How would you document this fall?

Multiple Choice. *Choose the correct answer or answers.*

43. Side effects of medication can cause serious problems in clients. _____ should be reported to the case manager immediately.

    a. unusual drowsiness

    b. disorientation and confusion

    c. falling and unsteady ambulation

    d. all of these

44. The most dangerous room in the house is the

    a. kitchen

    b. bedroom

    c. bathroom

    d. garage

45. If the home health aide's clothes start burning, the aide should

    a. run into the shower

    b. stop, drop, and roll

    c. use the fire extinguisher to put out the fire

    d. take off clothing

46. An easy-to-remember word to remind you how to operate a fire extinguisher is

    a. R-A-C-E

    b. F-A-S-T

    c. H-E-L-P

    d. P-A-S-S

47. For personal safety, a home health aide on entering a client's home should

   a. make note of the nearest exit from each room

   b. introduce herself then start to provide client care

   c. check the client's refrigerator for spoiled food

   d. take out the client's trash

Label the Diagram

48. Label the three elements of the fire triangle in the diagram (Figure 4–1) that are necessary to produce fire.

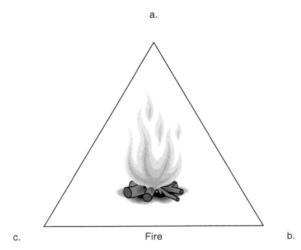

Figure 4–1

a. _____

b. _____

c. _____

PRACTICE SITUATIONS

Case 1

You arrive at your new client's home. Mr. Jaffe is sitting in the living room. Walking around the room are three chickens. From the looks of the house, they have been living there for some time. When you tell Mr. Jaffe that the chickens are causing a health hazard, he gets very upset and refuses to allow you to put them outside.

Questions

1. What will you do?

2. How can you give good care to your client and not have him become angry at you?

3. Should you call your case manager?

Case 2

You are assigned to care for Mrs. Peck. She has poor eyesight, uses a walker, and lives in a senior housing complex. There is a small passageway between furniture due to clutter and newspapers. Preparing lunch, you find outdated, sour milk and moldy food containers.

Questions

1. What safety issues are found in the home?

2. What should you do about conditions in the home?

3. As you are emptying the sour milk in the sink, Mrs. Peck starts shouting, "You're wasting my food." What response should you make?

CROSSWORD PUZZLE

Across

 3 safety problem found in home

 5 member of ambulance crew trained in basic life support

 7 number one cause of accidents in older adults

 9 maneuver used if person is choking

10 list of numbers to keep at telephone

Down

 1 leave building in case of fire/emergency

 2 device used to put out fires

 4 no smoking while wearing oxygen is an example of

 6 word to remember how to use a fire extinguisher

 8 what to do when fire occurs

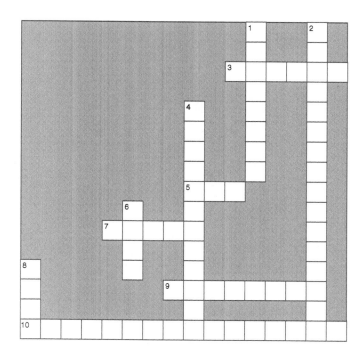

UNIT QUIZ

Multiple Choice. *Choose the correct answer or answers.*

1. Mrs. Dakus needs to wear her oxygen nasal cannula continuously due to COPD. Upon arrival to her home, you find her cooking at the gas stove while wearing her oxygen. What should you do?

   a. Shut off the oxygen immediately.

   b. Remind her it is not safe to use her gas stove while wearing her oxygen cannula. Request the client to leave the room and you will finish cooking her meal. Report the situation to your supervisor and case manager.

   c. Call 911.

   d. Call her physician and oxygen supply company.

2. Wheelchair-bound Mr. Rigby is forgetful. His clothes have burn marks on them from dropping ashes in the past. What safety guidelines should you follow?

   a. The client should smoke only while family or caregiver is present.

   b. Place a heavy, wide-rimmed ashtray or empty coffee can next to client while smoking to discard ashes in.

   c. Remove cigarettes and lighter from reach of client when caregiver not present and store outside client's bedroom.

   d. All of the above are correct.

3. Mr. Rigby is in his wheelchair and smoking a cigarette while you are changing his bed linens. You smell strong smoke and glance over to see his pant leg on fire. What should you do?

   a. Call 911 and wait for them to arrive.

   b. Use a fire extinguisher from the kitchen to extinguish the flames.

   c. Smother the flames with a blanket or sheet. Pull down and remove client's pants. Cool any reddened skin area with cool water. Notify case manager and family member.

   d. Call next-door neighbor for assistance. When he or she arrives, remove client from wheelchair, drop, and roll client on the ground.

4. Despite cerebral palsy, toddler Mohammed is able to get around his home with a walker. What age-appropriate safety tips should the family follow? Circle all that apply.

   a. Electrical extension cords should not be across the walking area, and safety plugs should be installed in unused electrical outlets.

   b. Pot handles should be turned inward on the stove and matches kept out of reach.

   c. Bicycle safety should be stressed, including wearing a helmet.

   d. Guns should be locked up and the preteen taught gun safety.

5. You arrive at Mrs. Rodriquez's home to find she's fast asleep in the living room chair with the TV on. The smoke alarm is going off. Upon entering the kitchen you see flames leaping from a pan and an empty bacon wrapper on the counter. You should first

   a. Call the client to wake her up.

   b. Call the fire department.

   c. Cover the pan with a lid or baking soda to smother the flames and turn off the burner.

   d. Use a Class A extinguisher to put out the fire.

6. How do you operate a fire extinguisher?

    a. Open the clear glass door, pull out the fire hose and turn on the handle at top of hose.

    b. Pull the pin at the top of the extinguisher, aim the nozzle toward the fire, squeeze the handle, and sweep the nozzle back and forth at the top of the flames.

    c. Call 911 for help.

    d. Pull the pin at the top of the extinguisher, aim the nozzle/outlet toward the fire, squeeze the handle, and sweep the nozzle back and forth at the base of the flames.

7. Safety tips for the home include all but

    a. Keep flammable items like gasoline, paint remover, and paint stored in proper containers in the basement near the heater.

    b. Water heater temperature should be set at 120 degrees Fahrenheit or less.

    c. Elderly clients should use a night-light due to decreased side vision.

    d. Place a smoke alarm on every level of the home.

8. If you are trapped by fire in a room you should

    a. Roll a rug or other materials and place it across the bottom of the door.

    b. Telephone for help if possible.

    c. Open a window, both top and bottom to allow air to enter and smoke to escape.

    d. All of the above are correct.

9. Tips for home safety for a client with dementia include

    a. Put safety knobs on the stove so the client cannot turn it on.

    b. Keep a night-light on at night to reduce confusion.

    c. Place additional locks on the outside door, preferably high up on the door.

    d. All of the above are correct.

10. The two groups that have the greatest risk of injury are

    a. infants and school-aged children

    b. school-aged children and preadolescents

    c. children and the elderly

    d. adolescents and school-aged children

11. Besides medication containers, childproof caps should be on

    a. milk and juice containers

    b. soft drink cans and bottles

    c. household cleaners

    d. none of these

12. Poor vision increases the risk of accidents because

    a. a person may not see objects in his or her path

    b. a person may not be able to see clearly and read medicine labels correctly

    c. warnings and labels can be misunderstood

    d. all of these

13. Personal safety tips for the home health aide include all but

    a. Do not wear long necklaces to avoid clients grabbing them and pulling your neck.

    b. Keep change in your pocket to be able to make a phone call in an emergency.

    c. Have your car keys ready when approaching your car.

    d. Wear makeup and flashy jewelry to brighten your client's day.

Fill in the Blanks. *Complete the following sentences with the correct word or words.*

14. _____ are physically active and willing to touch or taste almost anything. They may _____ on small objects.

15. _____ explore almost everything by looking, tasting, and touching. They have few fears and no judgment. Prevent _____ by turning pot handles inward on the stove.

16. Preteen children are _____ and not aware of dangers. They become involved in play and do not watch for hazards. Prevent injuries from bicycles by wearing a _____ _____ and teaching children how to safely _____ _____ _____.

17. Heavily influenced by their peers, _____ like to experiment, show off, and are careless. Accident prevention includes teaching about _____, burn prevention from careless _____ habits, and gun safety.

18. _____ have fewer accidents because learning is based on experiences. _____ may occur from careless use of outside fire, from overloaded electrical circuits, and from _____ in bed.

19. Old age causes many changes within the body: _____ are brittle, eyesight and hearing may fail. _____ may occur because labels cannot be seen due to poor eyesight.

UNIT 5   HOMEMAKING SERVICE

LEARNING OBJECTIVES

After studying this unit, you should be able to:

- List at least four tips used to plan and organize tasks
- Explain how to care for major home appliances
- Name three factors that determine the home health aide's cleaning plan
- List five cleaning tasks done daily
- List five cleaning tasks done weekly
- Describe the correct method for separating and disposing of garbage
- Identify at least four steps used in cleaning a kitchen
- Identify at least four steps used in cleaning the bathroom
- Explain how you would clean up a blood spill
- Discuss extra tasks that need to be done, if there are pets in the home
- List in order the linens used to make a regular bed using a soaker pad
- List five guidelines for bedmaking
- Describe the differences between a closed, open, occupied, and unoccupied bed
- Demonstrate the following:

  Procedure 1 Changing an Unoccupied bed

  Procedure 2 Changing an Occupied bed

TERMS TO DEFINE

- chronic obstructive pulmonary disease (COPD)
- closed bed
- dyspnea
- fanfold
- incontinent
- mitered corner
- occupied bed
- open bed
- unoccupied bed
- vomitus

APPLICATION EXERCISES

Short Answer/Fill in the Blanks. *Complete the following sentences with the correct word or words.*

1. Managing a household is like operating a daily 24-hour _____.

2. A professional home health aide must adapt to the _____ _____ of each job.

3. Labels should be _____ before using any cleaning product.

4. Wearing _____ will prevent skin irritations caused by soaps or detergents.

5. When handling the client's money, it is always important to get a _____.

6. If a client asks you to perform a task in a different way than you generally perform the task, you should _____ _____ _____ _____.

7. The home health aide should take a few minutes each morning to _____ the day's tasks.

8. Carrying cleaning supplies from _____ to _____ will help make the work go more quickly.

9. The order in which tasks are done is not always important. Plan the daily work around the _____ _____.

10. Sometimes it is possible to pair household tasks with _____ _____ _____, which helps save time and energy by avoiding many extra steps.

11. Cleaning tasks that need to be performed daily include:

    a. _____

    b. _____

    c. _____

    d. _____

    e. _____

12. Cleaning tasks that need to be performed weekly include:

    a. _____

    b. _____

    c. _____

    d. _____

    e. _____

13. Five cleaning tasks done on an occasional basis are:

    a. _____

    b. _____

    c. _____

    d. _____

    e. _____

14. When doing the laundry, first check the clothes for _____ and presoak them. Next, _____ clothes by colors and check _____ for tissues or change.

15. Loading the washing machine involves first putting _____ in the machine then _____ distribute clothes around the drum.

16. When cleaning the bathroom, start first with the _____. Place cleaner in bowl and with the _____ _____ _____ swish the solution around, paying special attention to the area under the rim of the bowl.

17. To avoid toilet clogs and odors, pour one cup of _____ _____ down the bowl weekly.

18. Clean the bathroom sink, countertops, shower, or tub with _____ to help kill the germs.

19. The bathtub needs to be cleaned thoroughly after each _____.

20. Best advice for cleaning the kitchen: work from the _____ to the _____ areas.

21. If blood or other body fluids are spilled on the floor, you must wear _____ and wipe up the spill with a solution of _____ part bleach to _____ parts water.

22. Cleaning supplies should be stored in a place that is safe from _____ and where disoriented _____ cannot reach.

23. Two purposes for changing a bed are:

   a. _____

   b. _____

24. List five linens generally needed to change a regular bed.

   a. _____

   b. _____

   c. _____

   d. _____

   e. _____

25. Guidelines for bed making include collect the linens in the _____ you will use them and hold soiled linens _____ from your uniform.

True or False. *Answer the following statements true (T) or false (F).*

26. T F   Never place anything metal in a microwave oven.

27. T F   Check the label before machine washing garments.

28. T F   Different colored clothing can be mixed together in the laundry.

29. T F   Mix ammonia and bleach products together for best results in cleaning the tub.

30. T F   Fluff the linens into the air while making a bed.

31. T F   Remove clothes from dryer promptly to avoid wrinkles.

Multiple Choice. *Choose the correct answer or answers.*

32. If the home health aide goes shopping for the client, the aide
    a. should make sure receipts are obtained for all purchases
    b. makes sure to buy the brands that the client requested
    c. gives the appropriate change to the client
    d. all of these

33. Things the home health aide can do to help organize household chores include
    a. making lists of needed supplies and chores to be performed
    b. performing whatever chore looks like it should be done
    c. always making sure the cabinets are closed
    d. wearing rubber gloves to protect hands

34. If the kitchen is kept clean and neat
    a. accidents are less likely to occur
    b. the meals will be easier to prepare
    c. germs are less likely to grow
    d. all of these

35. When the home health aide handles garbage from the household, the aide
    a. separates the garbage according to local guidelines
    b. double-bags the garbage
    c. wears gloves while handling the garbage
    d. all of these

36. The home health aide caring for the bathroom needs to remember to
    a. clean the toilet with bleach after each use
    b. clean the mirror after each use
    c. clean the bathtub with cleanser after each use
    d. all of these

37. While caring for an incontinent adult you should
    a. Double-diaper the client at bedtime to prevent leaks.
    b. Use adult briefs to save on bed linens and decrease unpleasant odor in the home.
    c. Use only a disposable soaker pad on the bed and leave the client's buttocks open to the air.
    d. Not use plastic protective bed covers to avoid suffocation.

38. Sally is making an occupied bed. This means that her client
    a. is in bed while Sally is changing the linens
    b. is sitting out of bed in a chair
    c. is out of bed and the linens are pulled to the top of the bed
    d. is out of bed and the linens are fanfolded to the foot of the bed

Documentation Exercises. *Read the following descriptions and provide documentation for each scenario.*

39. You are assigned to care for Mr. Smith. He needs a shower and a meal prepared. When you attempt to assist him to the shower, he tells you he does not feel like taking a shower and he is not hungry. You are aware that the client has a right to refuse care. How would you document his refusal?

40. Your client has an infectious disease. You must wash his dishes separately from other members of the household. How do you document this?

PRACTICE SITUATIONS

Case 1

You have been assigned to perform housekeeping chores at Mr. Santos's house. As you prepare to start cleaning, you notice cockroaches all over the kitchen. They are in the pantry, in the stove, and crawling on the cabinets. You had no idea that you would be asked to care for a mess like this.

Questions

1. What would you do first?
2. What area would you start to work in?

Case 2

You are cleaning the house and preparing a meal for Mrs. Kay. You have 4 hours and you need to clean the kitchen, wash the laundry, change the bed linens, clean the bathroom, and take Mrs. Kay for a walk. You also are aware that Mrs. Kay has severe arthritis and moves very slowly.

Questions

1. How will you organize your time?
2. In what order will you perform these tasks?

CROSSWORD PUZZLE

Across

1 bed made without the client in it, sheets fanfolded

3 unable to control urination

5 relating to health and cleanliness

6 shortness of breath

7 the steps taken to accomplish a particular task

Down

1 bed is made with the client in it

2 special corner made on bed to keep linens in place

4 to arrange in an orderly way

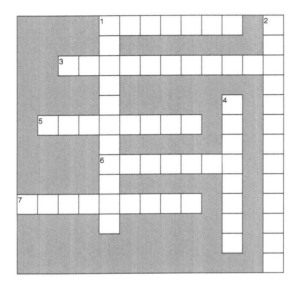

UNIT QUIZ

Matching. *Match each term with the correct definition*

1. ____ dryer
2. ____ washing machine
3. ____ dishwasher
4. ____ stove
5. ____ microwave
6. ____ refrigerator
7. ____ open bed
8. ____ mitered corner
9. ____ occupied bed
10. ____ unoccupied bed

a. put only recommended amount of soap in dispenser

b. clean outside and inside with mild soap or baking soda

c. wipe clean with wet cloth and soap. Rinse and wipe dry

d. clean the lint filter before or after each load

e. wipe up spills and grease at once. Wipe out oven with vinegar to remove surface dirt

f. put detergent in first, then distribute clothes evenly in the drum

g. the bed is being made without the client in it

h. the bed is being made with the client in it

i. special corner made on bed to keep linens in place

j. client is out of bed but the linens are fanfolded to the foot of the bed

Multiple Choice. *Choose the correct answer or answers.*

11. Mr. Wilkes, a chemotherapy patient, has vomitus on his bed linens. You should

    a. While wearing gloves, remove the linens, keeping them away from your body, and wash them as soon as possible.

    b. Wear gloves and disinfect the room with a 1:10 bleach solution.

    c. Gown, glove, and wear a mask when cleaning the room.

    d. Place contaminated linens into a trash bag for disposal.

12. Vomitus means

    a. loose control of your bowels or bladder, soiling clothes and surroundings

    b. material vomited and spit out from the mouth

    c. shortness of breath

    d. a blood spill from chemotherapy medication

13. Due to 25 years of smoking, Mr. Garcia now requires oxygen to breathe. His medical condition is called COPD or

    a. croupy obstinate peoples disease

    b. chronic orthostatic pulmonary disease

    c. crushing ortho penea disease

    d. chronic obstructive pulmonary disease

14. Mr. Garcia tells you he has "shortness of breath" when walking. You document in your notes

    a. Mr. Garcia reports he can't walk far.

    b. Mr. Garcia has dyspepsia when walking.

    c. Mr. Garcia reports dyspnea when walking.

    d. Mr. Garcia has diarrhea when walking.

15. Miss Anderson developed urinary incontinence after a stroke. This means

    a. she has a urinary tract infection

    b. she is unable to control urination

    c. she is bedbound and can't speak

    d. she needs to use a urostomy bag to collect urine

True or False. *Answer the following statements true (T) or false (F).*

16. T   F   Use a sharp knife to pry ice loose from freezer walls.

17. T   F   A cleaning plan should only be based on how much time the aide is in the home.

18. T   F   It is acceptable for the aide to perform extra chores for the client if given a few dollars by the client.

19. T   F   Cleaning products include soap, vinegar, and disinfectant cleaners.

20. T   F   Organizing your tasks and keeping lists of needed items for cleaning lightens the workload.

SECTION 2

Stages of Human Development

UNIT 6   INFANCY TO ADOLESCENCE

LEARNING OBJECTIVES

After studying this unit, you should be able to:
- Discuss issues dealing with pregnancy and childbirth
- Explain the term *bonding* of mother and infant
- Discuss Maslow's five basic needs
- List four abnormal conditions or diseases of infancy and early childhood
- Describe four common childhood illnesses
- List three signs of fetal alcohol syndrome
- List five safety checks for young children
- Describe three characteristics of toddlers
- List three characteristics of a preschool-aged child
- Discuss the seat belt requirements for infants and preschool children
- List three developmental tasks of adolescence
- Discuss smoking, use of illegal drugs, and alcohol abuse in adolescence
- Define child abuse
- List four behavioral patterns associated with abused children
- Discuss when and how to report cases of child abuse

TERMS TO DEFINE

- adolescence
- autism
- bonding
- cerebral palsy
- cesarean section
- child abuse
- conception
- cystic fibrosis
- developmental disability
- fetal alcohol syndrome (FAS)
- fetus
- gestation
- gestation period

- hierarchy
- learning disorder
- low birth weight
- obstetrician
- physiologic
- premature
- puberty
- self-actualization
- sexually transmitted disease (STD)
- sibling rivalry
- substance abuse
- sudden infant death syndrome (SIDS)

APPLICATION EXERCISES

Short Answer/Fill in the Blanks. *Complete the following sentences with the correct word or words.*

1. The fertilization of the female egg by the male sperm is called _____.

2. The _____ is the time from conception to birth.

3. Many complications of pregnancy and birth disorders may be prevented by _____.

4. _____ _____ is a surgical technique used to deliver the infant through an incision in the mother's uterus.

5. The process of _____ is an attachment of mother, father, and infant occurring after birth.

6. _____ and _____ are important in the first few months of the infant's life.

7. In psychologist Maslow's hierarchy, the first basic _____ need is for _____ and _____.

8. Maslow's highest human need is for _____ which is the _____ _____ _____ _____ _____ _____.

9. _____ is the infant's way of communicating that he or she needs something.

10. Infants weigh between _____ and _____ pounds at birth and have their birth weight usually _____ by age 1.

11. Children born with diseases or malformations need special _____ and _____ care.

12. Infants often treated in Neonatal Intensive Care Units (NICUs) are ones born before full term (before _____ _____ _____ _____) or weighing less than _____ _____ . They are called _____ infants.

13. In infants less than 1 year old, _____ _____ _____ _____ (SIDS) is a condition where a baby will stop breathing while asleep.

14. To prevent SIDS, doctors now recommend that babies be placed on their _____ when sleeping.

15. An apnea _____ may be placed on infants if a breathing disorder is suspected so that an alarm is sounded if the baby stops breathing.

16. Jealousy between older children and the new baby is called _____ _____.

17. Children sometimes need help adjusting to the _____ of big sister or big brother.

18. Older children need to _____ _____ _____ before touching baby to prevent the spread of _____ and _____.

19. Seven duties the aide may perform for the mother and the newborn are:

    a. _____

    b. _____

    c. _____

    d. _____

    e. _____

    f. _____

    g. _____

20. New mothers need plenty of rest, usually a nap in the _____ and one in the
    _____.

21. Visitors who have colds or similar infections should not _____ the baby.

22. Ages 1 and 2 are known as the _____ stage.

23. During the toddler stage, the child needs to be watched carefully because the toddler likes
    _____ _____ _____ _____.

24. Preschool age includes the ages _____ through _____.

25. _____ for achievements is better than punishments for _____.

26. Teenagers have a great need for _____.

27. During _____, the child is strongly influenced by the peer group.

28. During puberty, boys develop _____ on the face and under the arms.

29. Girls develop _____, _____, and _____ hair.

30. Between ages 10 to 15, young girls also begin to _____.

True or False. *Answer the following statements true (T) or false (F).*

31. T F Physical disciplines should never be given by the homemaker/home health aide.

32. T F Adolescents are hesitant to try new things.

33. T F Sex-related problems are especially common in adolescence.

34. T F It is estimated that 43 out of 1000 teenagers will become pregnant before they are 20.

35. T F Substance abuse is a serious problem. It has caused increased crime rate and has
          destroyed many families.

36. T F Religious practices sometimes determine the way birth control is practiced.

37. T F Teenagers are aware that alcohol is a dangerous drug.

38. T F If parents notice mood swings, red eyes, lethargy, overactivity, sniffling, or other
          unusual signs, they should seek help for their child.

39. T F According to the definition of a "legally responsible person," a home health aide
          working in the household would not be responsible for reporting abuse.

40. T F Abusive parents usually have not been raised by abusive parents themselves.

41. T F Life crises, such as job loss or debt, could cause abuse to a family member.

42. T F The home health aide should be aware of the signs of abuse. If the aide becomes aware
          of them, they need to be reported to the supervisor.

Matching. *Match the following common childhood illnesses or disorders with the correct definition.*

43. ____coxsackievirus

44. ____strep throat

45. ____bacterial conjunctivitis

46. ____croup

47. ____influenza

48. ____rotavirus

49. ____otitis media

50. ____attention-deficit/hyperactivity disorder

51. ____autism

a. childhood mental disorder marked by inattention, hyperactivity, and impulsivity

b. disorder involves withdrawal of the infant or child into a fantasy world of his or her creation

c. spread by direct contact with fecal material, nasal drainage, or saliva from infected person; rash appears on body, on hands, and on feet

d. bacterial infection passed by droplets in the air from nose and throat

e. redness of the white part of the eye, later pus appears

f. respiratory virus starts as cold symptoms followed by barky cough, awakening at night with difficulty breathing

g. symptoms include vomiting, diarrhea, abdominal cramps, and foul smelling stool

h. respiratory symptoms include congestion, cough, sore throat, body aches, headache, and fever

i. eardrum bulges due to increased amount of fluid and inflammation in the ear causing intense pain

Multiple Choice. *Choose the correct answer or answers.*

52. The newborn baby will need the home health aide to

    a. hold and cuddle him or her often

    b. feed him or her whenever he or she cries

    c. assist the mother with bathing the infant

    d. a and c only

53. The home health aide caring for a newborn infant with brothers and sisters needs to

    a. tell the children they cannot touch the baby

    b. encourage the children to help with the care of the infant

    c. allow the children to provide total care for the infant

    d. send the children outside to play while he or she cares for the infant

54. The home health aide assigned to care for a toddler needs to be aware that the toddler

    a. needs to be watched carefully because toddlers are very interested in everything

    b. is learning to talk and walk

    c. needs to be able to explore safely

    d. all of these

55. Adolescence is a difficult time because

    a. many physical and emotional changes are occurring in the youngster

    b. adolescents are just naturally difficult

    c. the adolescent needs special love and understanding

    d. a and c only

56. Teenage pregnancy is a problem because of

    a. sexually active younger teenagers

    b. an increase in sexually transmitted diseases

    c. lack of knowledge of birth control methods

    d. all of these

57. Substance abuse is

    a. the incorrect or misuse of prescription medications

    b. declining due to current drug laws

    c. the use of alcohol or drugs that results in poor treatment of the body

    d. not a significant problem in the United States due to drug awareness programs

58. Examples of maltreatment, child abuse, and neglect include

    a. exposure to lead poison from painted walls or furniture

    b. allowing children under 18 to drink alcohol or be given illegal drugs

    c. leaving children home alone in an apartment or house or locked in a room or car while the legally responsible adult is away

    d. all of the above

Documentation Exercises. *Read the following descriptions and provide documentation for each scenario.*

59. You are caring for an infant. He has several diarrhea stools. They are liquid and yellow in color. As you change his diaper, you notice his buttocks are slightly reddened. How would you document your observations?

60. Mrs. Petterson has a 3-year-old daughter and a set of twins. Her husband is working 12-hour shifts. You've been working two weeks assisting the family. Mrs. Petterson sleeps most of the time you are there and rarely eats meals you prepare. She talks to or holds the babies minimally. What should you document?

PRACTICE SITUATIONS

Case 1

You are caring for three children: Kathy, age 8; Johnny, age 6; and Judy, age 4. While you are bathing them, you notice several large bruises on Kathy. You ask her "What happened to cause these bruises?" Kathy looks down and says, "I fell." You are very concerned about this.

Questions

1. What would you do?
2. Would you talk to the other children?
3. Would you talk to the parents?
4. What are your responsibilities as a home health aide?

Case 2

When you are caring for your client, Mrs. Thyme and her infant, you hear loud talking in the back bedroom. You go to the room and you hear Mrs. Thyme's son and his friends. It sounds like they are taking drugs.

Questions

1. What can you do?
2. Can you go into the room?
3. Should you talk to Mrs. Thyme about your concerns?
4. If they are using illegal drugs, what must you do?

CROSSWORD PUZZLE

Across

4 an inherited condition that affects children's sweat glands, pancreas, and respiratory system

13 the time required from conception to birth

14 the time period following childhood when the body matures and reproduction becomes possible

Down

1 a full-term baby weighing less than 5 pounds

2 emotional or physical abuse of an individual under the age of 18

3 a process of attachment of mother, father, and infant happening immediately after birth

4 condition when there is impaired muscular power and coordination because of a lack of oxygen to the brain

5 sudden infant death syndrome

6 unborn child

7 sexually transmitted diseases

8 brothers and sisters

9 the period of physical and emotional development from early teens to young adulthood

10 the ability to resist certain diseases

11 an infant born before full term

12 occurs when a female egg is fertilized by a male sperm

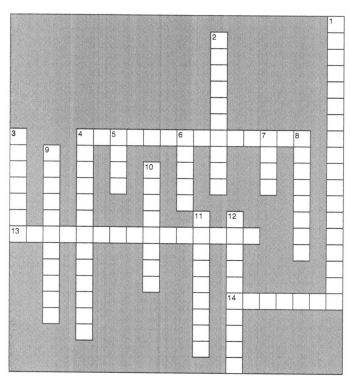

UNIT QUIZ

Matching. *Match each term with the correct definition.*

1. _____ bonding
2. _____ cesarean section
3. _____ conception
4. _____ prenatal care
5. _____ fetus
6. _____ sibling rivalry
7. _____ puberty
8. _____ obstetrician
9. _____ adolescence
10. _____ physiologic

a. surgical technique in which the infant is removed from the mother through an abdominal incision

b. fertilization of an egg by a sperm

c. care given during pregnancy

d. process of cuddling and fondling by one or both parents after a birth

e. unborn young

f. basic human need for food and shelter

g. health care provider who cares for pregnant women and delivers babies

h. children display jealousy of new family member

i. physical process of growing up: growth spurts, changing body size, and sexual organ development

j. period between ages 13 and 19 with broad developmental changes

Short Answer. *Complete the following sentences with the correct word or words.*

11. Four duties that a homemaker/home health aide might be expected to do for an infant are:

a. _____

b. _____

c. _____

d. _____

12. Five safety rules home health aides can follow while caring for young children are:

a. _____

b. _____

c. _____

d. _____

e. _____

13. List four abnormal conditions of infancy and early childhood.

a. _____

b. _____

c. _____

d. _____

Multiple Choice. *Choose the correct answer or answers.*

14. The homemaker/home health aide feels that the client (a new mother) is too weak to handle a baby alone. The homemaker/home health aide should

    a. realize that mothers can survive anything

    b. tell the mother to get more rest

    c. take the infant home (to the homemaker/home health aide's home) until the mother feels stronger

    d. notify the case manager immediately and factually report the concerns

15. You are assisting caring for Joseph, a 7-year-old child. He often sits and stares into space and rocks back and forth watching TV. Any change in routine causes him to wail and cry out or hide in his room. His medical problem is

    a. autism   c. cerebral palsy

    b. attention-deficit/hyperactivity disorder   d. cleft palate

16. Ten-year-old Mickey needs your assistance getting ready for school each morning. He wears special leg braces and shoes, uses crutches to walk short distances, and uses a wheelchair at school. He has

    a. autism   c. cerebral palsy

    b. attention-deficit/hyperactivity disorder   d. cleft palate

17. You are very careful feeding 9-month-old Angela. She has difficulty chewing and food gets trapped in her mouth due to a split in her lip and top of mouth. She is scheduled for surgery next month. Her disability is called

    a. autism   c. cerebral palsy

    b. attention-deficit/hyperactivity disorder   d. cleft palate

18. Miguel has a hard time sitting still at school. He often needs to get up and move around the classroom due to restless energy. His short attention span and impulsivity make it difficult to learn some subjects. Medication helps him with

    a. autism   c. cerebral palsy

    b. attention-deficit/hyperactivity disorder   d. cleft palate

19. Born at 30-weeks gestation with breathing problems, 6-week-old Sabrina is just coming home. She is attached to an apnea monitor due to high risk for

    a. infantile botulism   c. sudden infant death syndrome (SIDS)

    b. fetal alcohol syndrome   d. cystic fibrosis

20. Born to an alcoholic mother, Simon was only 4 pounds 6 ounces at birth. He has a small head, with flat face and narrow eyes. He remains fretful when handled at 6 months old and he needs coaxing to eat. The doctor says he has a weak heart. Simon shows signs of

    a. infantile botulism   c. sudden infant death syndrome (SIDS)

    b. fetal alcohol syndrome   d. cystic fibrosis

UNIT 7   EARLY AND MIDDLE ADULTHOOD

LEARNING OBJECTIVES

After studying this unit, you should be able to:

- Discuss three major decisions that a young adult will need to make during early adulthood
- List five preventive health checks that are recommended to be done before the age of 50 for women
- List five preventive health checks that are recommended to be done before the age of 50 for men
- Discuss three life changes that occur with middle adulthood
- List two reasons why a middle-aged adult should be involved in an exercise program or other social activities
- Discuss different personality traits that clients with disabilities often display
- Discuss recent changes in society and technology that have helped enhance the life of clients with special needs or disabilities

TERMS TO DEFINE

- bone density test
- cholesterol level
- colon
- Division of Vocational Rehabilitation (DVR)
- early adulthood
- electrocardiogram (ECG)
- empty nest syndrome
- mammogram
- menopause
- middle adulthood

- osteoporosis
- Pap smear
- preventive health measure
- prognosis
- prostate
- psychologist
- Special Olympics
- testicles
- thyroid-stimulating hormone (TSH) test

APPLICATION EXERCISES

Short Answer/Fill in the Blanks. *Complete the following sentences with the correct word or words.*

1. During early adulthood, one starts _____ his or her life and making _____ _____ that will affect the years to come.

2. The average age that individuals get married today is in the _____ _____ and the average age of mothers having their first baby is now _____.

3. During early adulthood, many individuals are interested in _____ _____ _____, joining various _____ _____, and doing something for their _____ or _____.

4. Health problems in early adulthood often accompany _____.

5. All persons should have a physical exam at least _____ _____ _____ _____ _____ as early detection of diseases often leads to a better _____ or outcome.

6. A woman should perform a breast self-examination _____; she should have a pelvic examination and a Pap smear performed _____.

7. A _____ examination should be performed on both men and women every five years after the age of 50.

8. The major threat to women's health today is not only breast cancer but _____ disease.

9. The major cause of death in men is _____ disease followed by _____ cancer, _____ cancer, and _____ cancer.

10. Middle adult years, ages _____ to _____, are ages when people are expected to be successful and productive.

11. Hormonal changes that occur during menopause may result in _____ _____, changes in _____ patterns, or increased _____.

12. When the grown children leave home, parents sometimes feel a loss. This is called _____ _____ _____.

13. _____ can make anyone old before his or her time.

14. One of the best exercises is _____.

15. As a home health aide, you need to encourage your clients to _____ if they are able to do so.

16. Individuals who keep themselves involved actively in some type of _____ _____ do better health wise, than those who become addicted to the _____ _____.

17. It is very difficult for middle-age adults to accept assistance with _____ _____ _____ (ADLs) and in some cases _____ assistance.

18. Two important needs of persons with disabling conditions are:

   a. _____

   b. _____

19. Psychologists tell us to center the attention of adults with disabilities on their _____ rather than their _____.

20. A major adjustment of most individuals is _____.

21. It is easier for a person with a disability or special needs to remain _____ and _____ active today due to specially equipped vans or public transit service.

22. Due to new laws and public awareness many restaurants and businesses have handicapped accessible ramps and _____ along with special accommodations for

   _____.

23. _____ _____ _____ _____ can set up a training program for _____ with special needs and assist with the costs.

Multiple Choice. *Choose the correct answer or answers.*

24. Hormonal changes during menopause can result in

   a. graying of the hair

   b. mood swings, hot flashes, increased problems sleeping

   c. the children leaving home

   d. all of these

25. The home health aide needs to be aware of the good effects of exercise, including

   a. problems with stretched muscles

   b. inactivity ages the body

   c. exercise can be called an antiaging pill

   d. exercise is very time-consuming

26. When caring for a client in this age group (25 to 65), the home health aide needs to remember that

   a. it is very difficult for these clients to accept assistance from others

   b. these clients are not very grateful at this age

   c. most middle-aged adults will expect you to do everything for them

   d. all of these

27. The client with a disability

   a. has the same emotional needs as healthy individuals

   b. generally likes to stay at home

   c. expects more assistance from the home health aide

   d. none of these

28. The main causes of health problems in young adults (25 to 45) include

   a. problems with arthritis

   b. problems associated with childbirth and accidental injuries

   c. cancer

   d. heart disease

Documentation Exercises. *Read the following descriptions and provide documentation for each scenario.*

29. You are caring for a 45-year-old client who is recovering from his first heart attack. He tells you that he does not know what to do: his health care provider has told him he must take a less stressful job. When you ask him if he is experiencing any pain, he says no but winces every time he moves in bed. How would you document this?

30. You are caring for a client who is recovering from a fractured leg. One of your duties is to assist her to the bathroom. You do this and she has no difficulty in ambulating with walker and your assistance. How would you document this?

PRACTICE SITUATIONS

Case 1

You wake up an hour later than usual. You do not know why your alarm clock did not go off at the proper time. You realize that you are going to be late to care for Mr. Howe. This causes you to be become very anxious.

Mr. Howe is a very particular client. He is recovering from a broken leg. He is an executive and worries all the time about schedules. He is angry that he is ill because it interferes with his work schedule. You call him and tell him you are running late. He grumbles but tells you to hurry up, he has a business client coming to his home to do business in about two hours.

Questions

1. What will you do to give good care without rushing?
2. Will you be able to carry out your duties?

Case 2

You are caring for Mrs. Lemmon. She is diabetic and has very poor eyesight. A car is in her driveway. She tells you that she drives to the store at least twice a week. You ask her how she can see to drive. She tells you she has been driving to the same store for more than 30 years and the car knows where to go.

Questions

1. Can you inform your case manager?

2. What can you do about this situation?

3. You know that no matter what you say or do, as long as that car is there and she has the keys, she will drive it. What legal responsibility do you have?

CROSSWORD PUZZLE

Across

1 direct examination of the interior of the sigmoid colon

8 x-rays of the female breasts used to determine whether a tumor is present

10 period between 25 and 45 years of age

Down

2 period between 45 and 65 years of age

3 value one places on oneself as a person functioning in society

4 to avoid illness before it starts

5 cessation of the monthly menstrual cycle

6 a medical technique whereby a sample of the vaginal cells are tested for cancer

7 the probable outcome of an illness

9 monthly self-exam recommended for males

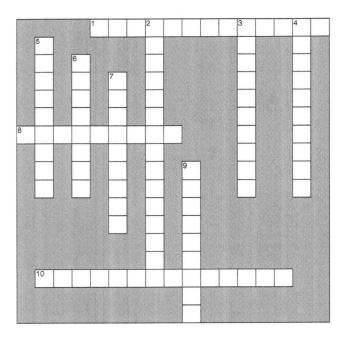

UNIT QUIZ

Short Answer/Fill in the Blanks. *Complete the following sentences with the correct word or words.*

1. Name three major decisions that a person will make during early adulthood.

   a. _____

   b. _____

   c. _____

2. List five preventive health checks recommended to be performed before age 50 for women.

   a. _____

   b. _____

   c. _____

   d. _____

   e. _____

3. List five preventive health checks recommended to be performed before age 50 for men.

   a. _____

   b. _____

   c. _____

   d. _____

   e. _____

4. Three lifestyle changes that occur with middle age are:

   a. _____

   b. _____

   c. _____

5. Two of the most important aspects of care of clients with disabilities are:

   a. _____

   b. _____

6. During early adulthood ages _____ to _____ the body usually heals quickly.

7. _____ _____ _____ are health recommendations to maintain a person's health and well-being and to prevent development of health problems.

8. Society places great demands on middle adulthood from _____ to _____ years of age.

9. The major cause of death in women today is _____ _____.

10. In men, the major cause of death is due to _____ _____.

Matching. *Match each term with the correct definition.*

11. _____ breasts   a. test that detects cervical cancer

12. _____ bone density test   b. test detects bone thinning/osteoporosis

13. _____ osteoporosis   c. softening of the bones

14. _____ cholesterol test   d. blood test detects cholesterol level

15. _____ electrocardiogram   e. test detects abnormal heart damage

16. _____ mammogram   f. monthly self-exam recommended for men

17. _____ menopause   g. self-exam recommended for women

18. _____ Pap smear   h. blood test measures thyroid hormone level

19. _____ testicles   i. test that detects breast tumors

20. _____ TSH   j. period of life when menstrual cycle stops

Multiple Choice. *Choose the correct answer or answers.*

21. Since having a diving accident at age 22 and developing quadriplegia, wheelchair-bound Michael, age 32, is known as a difficult patient. He is bitter, demanding, and critical of how his care is given, often calling the aides "stupid." What may account for this behavior?

a. It is difficult for individuals in this age bracket to adjust to needing assistance from others.

b. Michael is spoiled and doted on by his parents.

c. Michael is having difficulty accepting limited abilities, depressed over his condition, and unable to have an intimate relationship like his friends who visit.

d. a and c

22. Mary, age 46, has Down syndrome and mild multiple sclerosis. The aides assist her getting ready weekdays for her workshop job. You notice that she is fanning herself, her face is flushed, and she's more anxious than usual. She tells you she isn't sleeping well. You've noticed that her bed linens are quite twisted like she was tossing and turning and her pillow is damp. Mary's symptoms may be indicative of

a. myopathy

b. menopause

c. prostate problems

d. puberty

23. You are assisting Mrs. Cho as she recovers from a broken arm and leg due to an auto accident. Mrs. Cho was very active at her daughter's high school and soccer club but now her daughter is in college two states away. Mrs. Cho confides in you she doesn't know what to do with her future life as her children are all grown up. Mrs. Cho is experiencing

a. empty nest syndrome

b. baby blues

c. post-traumatic syndrome

d. menopause

24. Mr. Lightfoot has been hospitalized twice in six months due to COPD. He tells you he has no energy and just sits and watches TV. The physical therapist has written an exercise program and reviewed it with you. You encourage Mr. Lightfoot to walk in his apartment complex because

    a. Inactivity can make people old before their time.

    b. One of the best exercises is walking.

    c. Breathing and active range-of-motion exercises will help improve Mr. Lightfoot's strength and endurance.

    d. All of the above are correct.

25. Fifty-eight-year-old Mrs. Williams has suddenly gained custody of her son's twin 4-year-old girls, a 6-year-old son, and 13-year-old daughter. Mrs. Williams has arthritis and limited mobility and walks with a cane. You are assigned to help with child care. What can you do to *best* help this family?

    a. Offer to cook dinner each day, even though not on the care plan.

    b. Offer to baby-sit the twins in the evening.

    c. Encourage Mrs. Williams to join the "Parenting Again" program for grandparents at the local community center.

    d. Hold a fund-raising drive.

UNIT 8   OLDER ADULTHOOD

LEARNING OBJECTIVES

After studying this unit, you should be able to:

- Discuss the statistics regarding the older adult

- Name some developmental tasks of the older adult

- List two signs of depression

- Discuss leisure-time activities of the older adult

- Describe physical changes in the body systems due to the aging process

- List ways to assist the home health aide to work with client who are hard-of-hearing or who have low vision

- Discuss sleep changes affecting the older adult

- Discuss the home health aide's responsibility in monitoring pain in the client

- Discuss problems with medication administration with the older adult

- Demonstrate the following:
  Procedure 3   Inserting a Hearing Aid
  Procedure 4   Caring for an Artificial Eye
  Procedure 5   Assisting the Client with Self-Administered Medications

TERMS TO DEFINE

- accommodation
- analgesic
- antibodies
- arteriosclerosis
- arthroplasty
- arthroscopy
- atrophy
- auditory
- cataracts
- cerumen
- chronological age
- conjunctiva
- copius
- dementia

- endocrine glands
- estrogen
- floaters
- functional age
- glaucoma
- hypothyroidism
- immune system
- integumentary system
- intraocular pressure
- iris
- kyphosis
- labia
- melanoma
- nocturia

- orthopedic
- otosclerosis
- Parkinson's disease
- pelvis
- pendulous
- peripheral vision
- phantom pain

- presbycusis
- progesterone
- pupil
- referred pain
- transurethral resection (TURP)
- vertebrae

APPLICATION EXERCISES

Short Answer/Fill in the Blanks. *Complete the following sentences with the correct word or words.*

1. _____ is a normal process for all individuals.

2. _____ _____ means how long a person has lived while _____ _____ means how an individual is able to accomplish tasks of daily living.

3. In the United States _____ _____ persons are over age 65, about 13% of the population. By 2030, this number will double, resulting in one in every _____ Americans being over 65.

4. How a person meets and solves _____ in earlier life, determines the _____ in later maturity. Successful problem solving leads to _____ in life.

5. Five examples of developmental tasks of older adults are:

   a. _____

   b. _____

   c. _____

   d. _____

   e. _____

6. Name five habits frequently seen in people who age well.

   a. _____

   b. _____

   c. _____

   d. _____

   e. _____

7. _____ is a persistent sadness that makes it difficult to do day-to-day tasks.

8. Three clues that would lead the home health aide to believe the client is depressed are:

   a. _____

   b. _____

   c. _____

9. Many times depression goes _____ in older adults for a variety of reasons. If recognized early, depression can be readily _____.

10. Hearing ability gradually diminishes from the time a person is _____.

11. Presbycusis, the _____ _____ _____
_____ is quite common in the older adults.

12. Clients who are hard-of-hearing (HOH) may have nerve damage affecting the _____ nerve, a disorder called otosclerosis. This disorder occurs when the _____ of the inner ear harden and no longer carry _____ _____ in the usual fashion.

13. Impacted cerumen, known as _____ _____ is also a cause of hearing loss in older adults.

14. A home health aide working with an older adult who is hard-of-hearing should speak _____ and _____ while facing the person at eye level.

15. Vision changes in the older adult involve yellowing and thinner _____, glands produce less fluid with more evaporation, resulting in _____ _____, and older adults may complain of _____.

16. The _____ becomes smaller letting less light into the back of the eye, thus the older adult has difficulty with _____ _____ and depth of objects.

17. The older eye does not adapt quickly to changes in light level, requiring _____ _____ than the younger eye of a 20-year-old, with _____ causing anxiety and inability to concentrate.

18. Older adults lose _____ or side vision; the common term is called _____ _____.

19. Common eye diseases in the older adult are _____, clouding of the eye's lens and _____, which is due to the rise of intraocular pressure, which damages the optic nerve and if left untreated causes _____.

20. List five tips useful when working with a client who has difficulty seeing.

   a. _____

   b. _____

   c. _____

   d. _____

   e. _____

21. Caring for an artificial eye is important to:

   a. _____

   b. _____

22. Good nutrition in older adults may be affected by the following digestive system changes: less sensitive _____ _____, lack of some teeth or replacement _____, less saliva, causing problems breaking down foods and making the older adult _____, and problems with an inefficient _____ _____, causing choking on thin liquids.

23. List five tips for improving the nutrition status of the older adult client.

   a. _____

   b. _____

   c. _____

   d. _____

   e. _____

24. Urinary system changes involve the bladder and kidney size decreasing along with diminished muscle control, which may result in _____ (night urination), frequency, and leaking.

25. As one grows older, a person's muscles become weaker and sometimes _____.

26. _____ is minor surgery where the _____ surgeon repairs the knee joint using a scope to see inside of the knee.

27. Badly damaged or worn-out knees or hips require replacement, which is called

   _____.

28. As a person ages, _____ may occur when the padding between some of the _____, the small bones of the spinal column, shrinks, causing the vertebrae to bend forward.

29. Thinning of bone density caused by loss of bone mass and bone strength due to declining estrogen levels is called _____.

30. Mild exercise done regularly can improve _____, increase _____ mass, and improve _____.

31. Reproductive system changes in older females involve lowered _____ and _____ hormone levels, loss of pubic hair, shrinkage of the _____, reduced _____ size, and less lubrication of the cervix, with these changes making the person more vulnerable for infection and irritation.

32. Reproductive system changes in older males include reduced _____ hormones and reduced seminal fluid causing reduced sexual desire, atrophy of _____ with reduced sperm production, and enlargement of the _____ _____, causing problems with urination such as dribbling, frequent urination, and urinary tract infections.

33. The U.S. Centers for Disease Control and Prevention (CDC) reported in 1999 that people over 50 make up 13% of total HIV cases. More seniors are now being screened for _____ _____ _____ and _____ due to having sexual relations later in life.

34. Integumentary system changes include thinning of _____ like tissue paper, lack of fatty layer of skin, loss of hair, appearance of skin _____, and lack of oil production resulting in the skin becoming dry and _____ very easily.

35. The sense of _____ diminishes and older adults can _____ themselves and not even feel it.

36. Circulatory system changes involve hardening of the _____, less elasticity, and filling up of vessels with _____. The veins lose their ability to expand and contract resulting in diseases like _____ and congestive heart failure.

37. As we age, sleep is of _____ duration.

38. Nervous system changes involve _____ circulation of blood to the brain, gradual reduction of _____ _____, and slower transmission of _____.

39. Diseases of the nervous system include _____ (loss of memory) and _____ _____ (a degeneration of nerve cells in the brain that control muscle movement).

40. As a person ages, the ability to feel _____ diminishes, making the older adult very vulnerable to undiagnosed illness and _____.

41. Signs and symptoms suggestive of pain are increase in blood _____, sweating, facial _____, holding or squeezing a body part, _____ or vomiting, and crying, _____, or just not talking.

42. The home health aide should use the _____ _____ _____ when documenting the client's pain.

43. Name four types of pain.

    a. _____

    b. _____

    c. _____

    d. _____

44. The most common treatment of pain is with _____. There are mild pain relievers or _____ such as Tylenol or stronger pain relievers such as Percodan and Demerol.

45. Other nursing measures that might reduce pain are a _____, rest and relaxation, walking, _____ _____, or reading.

46. Today, many _____ are given to older adults to _____ diseases.

47. There are different types of medications such as _____ drugs, _____ drugs like aspirin, laxatives, and cough medicine, and vitamin supplements and _____ supplements such as Saint-John's-wort, ginseng, or glucosamine and chondroitin.

48. As a home health aide, you might be the first person to notice the signs of a drug reaction. List five signs you might observe.

    a. _____

    b. _____

    c. _____

    d. _____

    e _____

49. The nurse or pharmacist will prepare a _____ of medications prescribed and the time they are to be given each day. As a home health aide, you are _____ _____ to pour the client's medication from the bottle; the client needs to do this himself or herself.

50. Although home health aides do not administer medications, list five tasks you can assist with.

a. _____

b. _____

c. _____

d. _____

e. _____

Matching. *Match each term with the correct definition.*

51. _____ antibodies

52. _____ atrophy

53. _____ copious

54. _____ conjunctiva

55. _____ functional

56. _____ labia

57. _____ nocturia

58. _____ pendulous

59. _____ peripheral vision

60. _____ vertebrae

a. membrane that lines the eye

b. night urination

c. hanging loosely

d. small bones of the spinal column

e. cells that fight off invading organisms

f. side vision

g. large amount

h. how a person is able to accomplish tasks of daily living

i. wasting away

j. lips of vagina

True or False. *Answer the following statements true (T) or false (F).*

61. T   F   Urinary incontinence is always a problem in older women.

62. T   F   Referred pain is pain felt farther away from the originating area.

63. T   F   Blindness in older adults is a frequent problem in the late 80s.

64. T   F   Common cancers in women are lung, breast, and ovarian cancer.

65. T   F   Dry eyes may be relieved with the use of natural tears eyedrops.

66. T   F   The bladder elongates in older adults causing frequent nighttime bathroom trips.

67. T   F   Skin tears occur in older adults due to decreased elasticity and fatty skin layer.

68. T   F   Depression is easily recognized but hard to treat in older adults.

69. T   F   Osteoporosis causes many fractures in adult men and women.

70. T   F   Constipation in older adults is related to decreased fluid and fiber intake.

Multiple Choice. *Choose the correct answer or answers.*

71. Two common threads in most older adults' lives are

a. change and loss

b. divorce and remarriage

c. supporting younger children and grandchildren

d. poor eyesight and leaking bladders

72. The benefits of exercise to the older adult include

a. improved digestion

b. decreased bone density

c. increased muscle mass

d. improved sleep

73. Healthy leisure time activities include all but
    - a. playing cards with friends
    - b. traveling in a motor home
    - c. attending the Senior Center
    - d. sitting in recliner watching TV all day

74. The phenomenon of daughters caring for their aging parents and their own children is called
    - a. sandwich generation
    - b. baby boomers
    - c. generation X
    - d. boxing generation

75. Age-related mental changes the home health aide can expect to see in elderly clients include
    - a. depression
    - b. dementia
    - c. reminiscence about earlier times
    - d. all of these

76. Persons who have not successfully solved problems may show signs of
    - a. anxiety
    - b. depression
    - c. inability for personal growth
    - d. decreased bone growth

77. Increasing life expectancy to well beyond 80 is the result of all but
    - a. better public health measures
    - b. advances in medical care and technology
    - c. improvements in living conditions
    - d. air transportation

78. Which sense affects both taste and appetite?
    - a. smell
    - b. hearing
    - c. vision
    - d. touch

79. The home health aide preparing meals for the older adult
    - a. needs to include well-cooked food
    - b. should include a lot of red meat
    - c. should offer a variety of foods, including fruits, vegetables, and carbohydrates
    - d. none of these

80. The home health aide assists in hearing aid care by
    - a. checking the earmold to see if it is plugged with wax
    - b. checking that the batteries are working
    - c. assisting the client in inserting the earmold in the ear canal
    - d. all of the above

Documentation Exercises. *Read the following descriptions and provide documentation for each scenario.*

81. You enter your client's apartment. Your client, Mrs. Stone, is a 45-year-old woman recovering from a stroke. The first thing you see is her medicine box lying on the floor with all the pills scattered. You ask her what happened. She tells you she does not know. She cannot remember what medicines she has taken. You immediately notify your case manager. How would you document this occurrence?

82. You are caring for an 80-year-old client who is very arthritic and a little confused. While you are in the bathroom cleaning the tub, you hear her fall from her chair. After you examine her, you call for assistance because her leg does not look right to you. Document this.

PRACTICE SITUATIONS

Case 1

Mrs. Klein is your client. She is very sweet and very cooperative except in one area. She is constantly dribbling urine. You have asked her to wear adult incontinent products, but she refuses. She is unsteady on her feet, and you are worried about her falling by slipping in the urine.

Questions

1. What alternatives can you think of?

Case 2

You are looking forward to meeting your new client, Mrs. Donald. However, when you arrive at her home, you encounter two large dogs. They are not going to let you in. Before you left home, you tried to call Mrs. Donald, however, she has no telephone.

Questions

1. What do you do?

2. She cannot hear you and does not know what time you are coming. What choices do you have?

CROSSWORD PUZZLE

Across

1 large amount

3 pain experienced with loss of limb

4 urinary frequency during nighttime

6 eye disease caused by increased intraocular pressure

8 severance of something

9 progressive mental deterioration caused by organic brain disease

10 loss of bone density

11 usually refers to persons over the age of 65

Down

1 membrane that lines the eye

2 a mental state characterized by loss of hope, feelings of rejection, and generalized sadness

5 loss of voluntary control of bladder muscles, causing uncontrolled urination

7 clouding of the lens of the eye

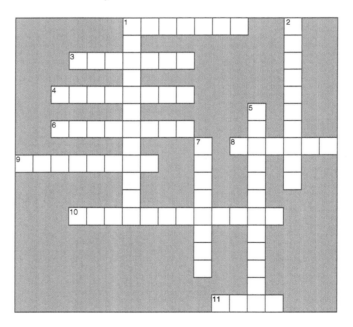

UNIT QUIZ

Multiple Choice. *Choose the correct answer or answers.*

1. Physical examinations are done

   a. to maintain wellness

   b. to detect some diseases early like cancer and heart disease

   c. as a good approach to preventive medicine

   d. to make sure employees are able to perform certain duties that are in their job description

2. The client who is totally nonambulatory (unable to walk) needs

    a. no special treatment because he or she is always in one place

    b. to be positioned at least every two hours to prevent bedsores

    c. to be checked frequently for constipation

    d. diversions such as radio, TV, or frequent visitors to prevent boredom

3. Mr. Johnson refuses to have his prescription refilled. A home health aide's responsibility is to

    a. report this to the case manager   c. call the doctor

    b. encourage him to use his wife's medication   d. do nothing

4. Change in the elderly

    a. is a frequent occurrence   c. may result in depression

    b. involves losses   d. all of these

5. Because of less hormone production, there is an increase in

    a. parathyroidism   c. diabetes

    b. testosterone   d. hypothyroidism

6. Preventive health measures for the older adult involve receiving

    a. flu vaccine   c. screening for HIV

    b. pneumonia vaccine   d. all of the above

7. Respiratory system changes include

    a. decreased elasticity of the lungs   c. diminished breathing capacity

    b. thickening of lung secretions   d. all of the above

Matching. *Match the medical term with the correct definition.*

8. _____ arteriosclerosis

9. _____ arthroplasty

10. _____ dementia

11. _____ cataracts

12. _____ glaucoma

13. _____ hypothyroidism

14. _____ melanoma

15. _____ osteoporosis

16. _____ Parkinson's disease

17. _____ transurethral resection

a. replacement of joint

b. loss of vision due to raised intraocular pressure

c. decrease in bone mass

d. malignant skin cancer

e. hardening of the arteries

f. loss of memory

g. degeneration of brain cells that control muscles

h. prostate surgery

i. severe thyroid deficiency

j. clouding of the eye's lens

Short Answer/Fill in the Blanks. *Complete the following sentences with the correct word or words.*

18. Miss Johnson has sprained her ankle. Her pain has a sudden onset, is well defined, and will run a short course. This is an example of _____ pain.

19. Mr. Garcia takes Percodan and has seen many specialists in three years for his back pain. Three sessions of physical therapy have brought little relief. He wears a back brace and is easily fatigued. He is experiencing _____ pain.

20. The home health aide is one of the people who sees the elderly client regularly. The aide has the opportunity to identify _____ that could be significant.

21. Granny Smith lives alone. Her freezer is full of meat, while the refrigerator has stale milk and moldy bread. She complains of being hungry. She has worn the same clothes your past two visits, even though you helped her bathe and change clothes. She repeats many of the same phrases each visit. You suspect she may have _____ and report your concerns to her case manager.

22. Mrs. Forrest has high blood pressure, arthritis, and uses many medications. While bathing her, you observed bruises on her arms. She complains of being dizzy when getting up from the tub and states she's tired and weak from not sleeping this weekend. These are possible symptoms of a _____ _____ and you should immediately notify your case manager.

23. Three physical changes that occur during the older years are:

    a. _____

    b. _____

    c. _____

24. The emotional changes that may occur in late adulthood are:

    a. _____

    b. _____

25. List three ways home health aides can assist older adults with medication administration.

    a. _____

    b. _____

    c. _____

SECTION 3

Preventing the Spread of Infectious Disease

UNIT 9   PRINCIPLES OF INFECTION CONTROL

LEARNING OBJECTIVES

After studying this unit, you should be able to:

- Name three different types of microorganisms
- List signs and symptoms of an infection
- Distinguish between an infection and an inflammation
- Explain the chain of infection
- Explain the differences between disinfection, aseptic technique, and sterilization
- Describe infection control practices
- List six ways diseases are carried
- Describe standard precautions and when used
- Describe the three types of transmission-based precautions and when used
- List five requirements of OSHA and CDC that affect home health aides
- List signs and symptoms and nursing care for a client with tuberculosis
- Discuss three types of hepatitis and the differences between them
- Discuss how a person can become infected with HIV
- Describe the three different stages of HIV/AIDS
- Discuss symptom-specific nursing care for clients with AIDS
- Name the single most effective precaution to prevent the spread of infections
- List five examples of when aides must wash their hands
- Explain the purpose of each procedure
- Demonstrate the following:
  Procedure 6   Handwashing
  Procedure 7   Gloving
  Procedure 8   Putting on and Removing Personal Protective Equipment
  Procedure 9   Collecting Specimen from Client on Transmission-Based Precautions

TERMS TO DEFINE

- acquired immunodeficiency syndrome (AIDS)
- airborne
- antibiotic-resistant
- antimicrobial
- aseptic techniques
- bacteria
- conjunctivitis

- contact precautions
- contaminated
- disinfection
- droplet precautions
- fungi
- germs
- hepatitis A, B, C
- herpes zoster (shingles)
- Highly Active Anti-Retroviral Therapy (HAART)
- human immunodeficiency virus (HIV)
- incident report
- incubation period
- infection
- infectious disease
- inflammation
- isolation
- jaundice
- Kaposi's sarcoma
- methicillin-resistant *Staphylococcus aureus* (MRSA)
- microorganisms
- nosocomial infection
- Occupational Safety and Health Administration (OSHA)
- OraQuick
- pathogens
- *Pneumocystis carinii* pneumonia
- portal of entry
- protozoa
- reservoir
- rickettsiae
- severe acute respiratory syndrome (SARS)
- standard precautions
- sterile
- susceptible host
- transmission-based precautions
- tuberculosis
- U.S. Centers for Disease Control and Prevention (CDC)
- vancomycin-resistant enterococcus (VRE)
- virus

APPLICATION EXERCISES

Short Answer/Fill in the Blanks. *Complete the following sentences with the correct word or words.*

1. The invasion of the body by disease-producing organisms is called an _____.

2. Microorganisms are so small they can only be seen by the use of a _____.

3. Disease-producing microorganisms are called _____.

4. Germs spread rapidly from one part of the body to _____.

5. Signs of a client having an infection are _____ and _____, fatigue, loss of appetite, _____ from infected area, _____ , pain or _____, nausea and vomiting, _____, or a skin rash.

6. Inflammation of a body part may have similar signs but does not have a _____ in the area.

7. Infectious diseases can be spread through various routes: _____, animal and _____ carried, contact or _____ carried, prenatal, food on food, soil and _____ carried.

8. The best defense against the spread of _____ is good infection control.

9. If a client develops an infection while being hospitalized, this type of infection is called
   _____ _____.

10. Articles that are free of all living things are _____. If the article has any
    possibility of having germs on it, it is considered to be _____.

11. The process of _____ completely destroys microorganisms on objects.

12. Sterilized supplies must be handled in a special way to prevent them from becoming
    _____.

13. The process of destroying disease-producing organisms by the use of chemicals is called
    _____.

14. If two people are using the same stethoscope, the earpieces must be cleaned with
    _____ _____ between uses along with the diaphragm of the
    stethoscope between patients.

15. Three airborne diseases are:

    a. _____

    b. _____

    c. _____

16. A home health aide needs to understand how to keep pathogens from _____.

17. The spread of disease from one person to another is called _____
    _____.

18. Aseptic techniques are used to _____ _____
    _____ _____ _____.

19. Four ways that diseases can be transmitted are:

    a. _____

    b. _____

    c. _____

    d. _____

20. Three diseases carried by food are:

    a. _____

    b. _____

    c. _____

21. _____ _____, _____, and
    _____ are diseases that are transmitted to humans from contaminated
    drinking water.

22. Two diseases that are transmitted to unborn children by the mother are _____
    and _____.

23. When a person steps on a rusty nail, there is a possibility he or she could contract
    _____.

24. Hepatitis is a _____ infection that mainly affects the _____.
    The three main types are hepatitis _____, _____,
    _____.

25. Classic signs and symptoms of hepatitis are _____, _____,
    abdominal _____, loss of _____, and _____.

26. Hepatitis _____ is the more serious type of hepatitis and could lead to complications that may cause _____ cancer or _____ of the liver. This disease can be treated with a variety of _____.

27. Hepatitis C is caused by _____ _____ virus and is spread through _____ _____ of intravenous drug users, needle-stick injuries at work, or an infant can contract the infection while in utero, if the _____ is infected.

28. A chronic disease that remains in the bloodstream, hepatitis C will eventually destroy the person's _____ and is the leading cause for liver _____ in the United States.

29. The home health aide may get _____ to prevent acquiring the hepatitis B virus; the vaccine is divided into _____ injections over a six-month period.

30. Home health aides taking care of clients with hepatitis should give them good _____ and _____ care.

31. Tuberculosis (TB) is an _____ disease and the incidence of TB is on the _____.

32. Individuals most susceptible to TB are persons who live in _____ _____, have _____ _____, are substance _____, are under _____, and lack _____ _____.

33. An aide taking care of a client with TB will need to use _____ _____, especially when handling the client's sputum and nasal secretions.

34. Home health aides need to be checked _____ for TB by having a TB skin test. If the home health aide tests positive for TB, he or she needs to get a _____ _____.

35. Four signs of TB are:

   a. _____

   b. _____

   c. _____

   d. _____

36. It is important for the client with TB to get plenty of _____ and take _____ as prescribed on schedule, otherwise the effects of the drugs will be _____.

37. Three childhood communicable diseases are:

   a. _____

   b. _____

   c. _____

38. An _____ contracting a childhood disease is affected more seriously than a _____.

39. An aide caring for a sick child needs to practice good infection control techniques to avoid becoming _____ _____.

40. When people are ill, the person's body is so busy fighting one illness it _____ fight off other germs.

41. Germs can enter the body in many ways. Four ways are:

    a. _____

    b. _____

    c. _____

    d. _____

42. Guidelines for working with clients with infectious disease come from two government agencies: U.S. Centers for Disease Control and Prevention (_____) and Occupational Safety and Health Administration (_____).

43. Accredited home health agencies must follow the following OSHA employer guidelines:

    a. _____

    b. _____

    c. _____

    d. _____

    e. _____

44. An _____ _____ is filled out by a home health aide to report accidental needle-sticks or sharp instrument finger pricks or any accident in the client's home.

45. The home health aide's _____ are the most common source of carrying infection.

46. The most important procedure in controlling the spread of disease is _____ _____.

47. To dry the hands, use of _____ _____ _____ is best; the use of cloth towels can _____ germs when reused.

48. List six times hands should be washed while in the client's home.

    a. _____

    b. _____

    c. _____

    d. _____

    e. _____

    f. _____

49. Standard precautions provide guidelines for _____; personal protective equipment use: _____, _____, _____, _____; client care equipment; _____ _____; _____ _____; and safe needle use.

50. _____ _____ _____ are used when the pathogen that is causing an infection is highly contagious.

51. Three types of transmission-based precautions are:

    a. _____

    b. _____

    c. _____

52. Contact precautions involve:

    a. _____

    b. _____

    c. _____

    d. _____

    e. _____

53. Two organisms seen in home health care that are resistant to antibiotics are:

    a. _____

    b. _____

54. Five common infection control practices most people practice in daily living include:

    a. _____

    b. _____

    c. _____

    d. _____

    e. _____

55. A diagnosis of HIV is made through a _____ _____. Today there is a home test called _____, which can be done at home if a person thinks he or she might have been infected with the virus.

56. Acquired immunodeficiency syndrome (_____) is a severe immunologic disorder caused by the _____ _____ _____ transmitted by _____ _____ and drug users _____ _____.

57. A blood test called the _____ _____ is done to monitor the progress of the disease. Once the count goes below _____ then the diagnosis of AIDS is given.

58. Signs of a lower CD4 count are:

    a. _____

    b. _____

    c. _____

    d. _____

    e. _____

59. Since 1995, in the United States, the number of people dying from AIDS has dropped from 50,000 per year to less than 17,000. Many doctors believe the reduction in deaths is due to _____ (Highly Active Anti-Retroviral Therapy), the most successful drug regimen to date.

60. A rare form of skin cancer occurs in the later stages of AIDS called _____ _____. Other later signs are _____, brain cancer, and _____ _____ _____.

61. List five tips for working with AIDS clients.

a. _____

b. _____

c. _____

d. _____

e. _____

True or False. *Answer the following statements true (T) or false (F).*

62. T F Wash fresh fruits and vegetables before eating or storing them.

63. T F After being stored in the cabinet for several weeks, can tops do not need to be cleaned off before opening.

64. T F We cannot tell whether people have an infectious disease by looking at them.

65. T F It is unnecessary to use standard precautions if you know the client is not contagious.

66. T F The client who is feeling isolated or depressed may feel more depressed when the home health aide uses protective barriers such as masks and gowns.

67. T F Isolation means the client is kept away from others in the household.

68. T F It is unnecessary to wear gloves when emptying a bedpan.

69. T F You can wear the moisture-resistant gown only once.

70. T F All articles used by the client in isolation can be shared with the family.

71. T F If blood is spilled on the floor, a preparation of 1 part bleach and 10 parts water must be used to clean it up.

72. T F All contaminated materials from the client's room must be discarded by using a special paper or plastic bag and either burning it or placing it in a covered garbage container.

73. T F The client's dishes must be washed separately in hot, soapy water rinsed and air-dried.

Matching. *Match each term with the correct definition.*

74. _____ bacteria

75. _____ fungi

76. _____ protozoa

77. _____ pathogens

78. _____ viruses

79. _____ rickettsiae

a. microorganisms that can live only on living cells

b. tiny one-celled microorganisms

c. disease-producing microorganisms

d. microscopic organisms that multiply rapidly

e. a microorganism that lives on lice, ticks, fleas, and mites

f. include yeasts and molds

Documentation Exercises. *Read the following descriptions and provide documentation for each scenario.*

80. You are caring for a client with TB. You are requested to obtain a sputum specimen. You follow the procedure for collecting a sputum specimen. Document the procedure.

81. You are caring for an AIDS client. While you are caring for him, he vomits on the bathroom floor. You clean up the vomitus following correct procedure. Document this occurrence.

Multiple Choice. *Choose the correct answer or answers.*

82. The home health aide can help prevent the spread of disease by
    a. keeping hands clean
    b. covering nose when sneezing
    c. maintaining good health
    d. all of these

83. Caring for food properly can help prevent the spread of disease. Some things the home health aide can do include
    a. washing fruits and vegetables before eating them
    b. rinsing off the can tops before opening them
    c. cooking meats properly
    d. all of these

84. The home health aide needs to wear gloves when
    a. preparing foods for the client
    b. making the bed of a client
    c. handling body fluids
    d. all of these

85. The home health aide's hands need to be washed
    a. before providing care to a client
    b. before and after putting on gloves
    c. after making the bed
    d. a and b only

Short Answer

86. Refer to Figure 9–1. Describe why each item is important in preventing the spread of infection.

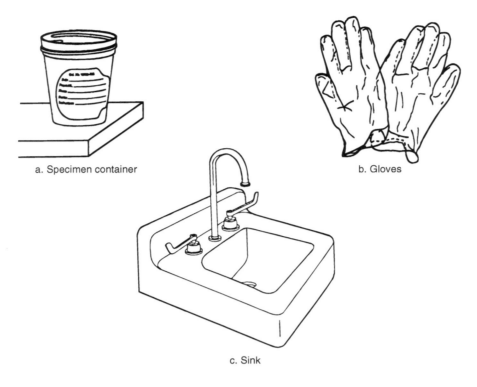

a. Specimen container

b. Gloves

c. Sink

Figure 9–1

a. _____

b. _____

c. _____

PRACTICE SITUATIONS

Case 1

You are caring for a teenage girl who has TB and is still contagious. When caring for her, you are required to use isolation precautions. However, she has several friends who are very un-cooperative. Every time your back is turned, they are in her room. You have asked the parents for assistance. But as soon as they leave, the girls are back.

Questions

1. What can you do?

2. How can you keep your client isolated?

Case 2

Your client has measles. You have never had the measles.

Questions

1. How would you care for your client without developing the measles?

2. What precautions would you use?

CROSSWORD PUZZLE

Across

1 lung disease

9 type of standard precautions

10 microorganisms capable of causing disease

11 microorganisms that can cause disease and live on lice, ticks, fleas, and mites

12 microorganism that lives and grows by feeding on living cells

17 invasion of pathogenic organisms causing infection

18 organisms not visible to the naked eye that can cause disease

Down

2 contains pathogens that may lead to infection

3 government agency responsible for employer health regulations

4 procedure whereby client is kept away from others to prevent spread of a contagious disease

5 inflammation of the liver

6 microorganisms causing disease

7 yellowish color of skin, eyes, and mucous membranes

8 hospital acquired infection

13 free of pathogens

14 one-celled microorganisms

15 diseases that can spread from one person to another

16 hostile entry into another area or place

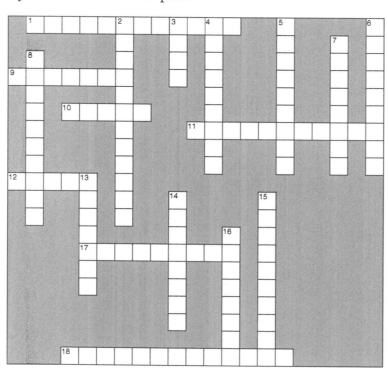

UNIT QUIZ

Multiple Choice. *Choose the correct answer or answers.*

1. A microorganism is a

    a. small, living plant or animal that can be seen only with a microscope

    b. germ that can cause disease

    c. certain insect

    d. plant that lives on other plants or animals

2. A microorganism that can cause an infection is called a

    a. nonpathogen   c. host

    b. germ   d. pathogen

3. Signs of infection include all of the following except

    a. fever   c. headache

    b. redness and swelling of a body part   d. discharge or drainage

4. Microorganisms can be transmitted by

    a. food, water, animals, and insects   c. personal care and hygiene equipment

    b. eating and drinking utensils   d. all of these

5. The practices used to prevent the spread of pathogens from one person or place to another are called

    a. sterilization   c. contamination

    b. medical asepsis   d. disinfection

6. A home health aide needs to understand how to keep germs from

    a. spreading   c. shedding

    b. sharing   d. reproducing

7. The most important way of controlling the spread of illness is by

    a. vaccination   c. sterilization

    b. disinfection   d. handwashing

8. An example of an airborne illness is

    a. tuberculosis   c. AIDS

    b. dysentery   d. food poisoning

9. The home health aide uses these measures daily to prevent the spread of infection

    a. isolation measures   c. contact precautions

    b. standard precautions   d. disinfection techniques

10. To prevent the spread of infection, disposal of soiled tissues and dressings involves

    a. burning the items in an incinerator   c. double-bagging for trash disposal

    b. spraying the items with disinfectant   d. pouring 1:10 bleach solution on items

11. Mr. Luongo has lung cancer and is receiving chemotherapy. While assisting him out of the tub, you hear him complain about having an itchy rash on his chest. You check his chest and see the rash, suspecting he may have

    a. shingles   c. measles

    b. impetigo   d. scarlet fever

12. Mr. Parker is a 56-year-old migrant worker. He has been struggling with alcoholism for several years. You are caring for his wife who has multiple sclerosis. He comes home early from work, complaining about shortness of breath and coughs repeatedly into tissues, which you note have a rusty appearance. You are concerned about his wife and you catching

    a. meningitis   c. tuberculosis

    b. bronchitis   d. AIDS

13. What should you tell Mr. Parker about his cough?

    a. He should wash his hands after handling tissues.

    b. Rusty sputum is a sign of tuberculosis, a communicable disease.

    c. He should get an appointment with his health care provider immediately.

    d. All of the above are correct.

14. Which infection control techniques would you follow while caring for Mrs. Parker?

    a. standard precautions   c. droplet precautions

    b. isolation precautions   d. contact precautions

15. Client care techniques to reduce infection include

    a. wiping off diaphragm of stethoscope with alcohol wipe

    b. holding soiled bed linens away from aides' clothes

    c. double-bagging of soiled dressings

    d. all of the above

Short Answer/Fill in the Blanks. *Complete the following sentences with the correct word or words.*

16. List five aspects of handwashing.

    a. _____

    b. _____

    c. _____

    d. _____

    e. _____

17. Protective barriers used in standard precautions include:

    a. _____

    b. _____

    c. _____

    d. _____

18. Blood spills need to be cleaned up using a preparation of _____ part bleach to _____ parts water with fresh solution prepared _____.

19. The purpose of putting on and removing personal protective equipment is to:

    a. _____

    b. _____

20. The three types of transmission-based precautions are:

    a. _____

    b. _____

    c. _____

Matching. *Match each term with the correct definition.*

21. _____ host   a. source of infection

22. _____ portal of entry   b. place germs live and thrive

23. _____ source   c. germ leaves the reservoir

24. _____ nosocomial   d. person or place where germ may live

25. _____ reservoir   e. infection acquired while hospitalized

SECTION 4

Understanding Health

UNIT 10   FROM WELLNESS TO ILLNESS

LEARNING OBJECTIVES

After studying this unit, you should be able to:

- Discuss wellness
- Make a distinction between an emotional disorder and an internal disorder
- Define disability
- Explain why vital signs are measured
- List the factors that affect vital signs
- Identify abnormal and normal temperature ranges
- Measure body temperature using different types of thermometers
- Identify various sites for taking a pulse
- Explain the normal range of pulse for different age groups
- Describe characteristics of normal and abnormal pulses
- Describe the normal rate of respiration in an adult
- Describe characteristics of normal and abnormal respirations
- Describe the normal and abnormal ranges for blood pressure
- Name the pieces of equipment used to take blood pressure
- Describe the two-step method of taking blood pressure
- List requirements for accuracy in measuring height and weight
- Distinguish between the different levels of unconsciousness
- Discuss nursing measures that need to be done for clients who are unconscious
- Discuss hypothermia and hyperthermia
- Demonstrate the following:
  Procedure 10   Taking a Tympanic (Ear) Temperature
  Procedure 11   Taking an Oral Temperature (Digital Thermometer)
  Procedure 12   Taking an Axillary Temperature
  Procedure 13   Taking a Rectal Temperature (Digital Thermometer)
  Procedure 14   Taking a Radial Pulse
  Procedure 15   Taking an Apical Pulse
  Procedure 16   Counting Respirations
  Procedure 17   Taking Blood Pressure
  Procedure 18   Measuring Weight and Height

TERMS TO DEFINE

- afebrile
- apical
- apnea
- blood pressure
- brachial
- bradycardia
- Celsius/centigrade
- Cheyne-Stokes respiration
- contracture
- diastolic
- disability
- dyspnea
- exhalation
- Fahrenheit
- febrile
- hypertension
- hyperthermia
- hypotension
- hypothermia
- inhalation
- orthostatic hypotension
- palpate
- pulse
- rales
- respiration
- sign
- sphygmomanometer
- stertorous
- symptom
- systolic
- tachycardia
- tympanic
- vital signs

APPLICATION EXERCISES

Short Answer/Fill in the Blanks. *Complete the following sentences with the correct word or words.*

1. _____ is the passing of traits and other individual differences.

2. Environment is the sum total of the circumstances, conditions, and _____ that affect the growth of an organism.

3. Both _____ and _____ contribute to an individual's development.

4. The role of the home health aide is involved in _____ the environment for the client.

5. The human body can adapt to many _____.

6. The smallest structural unit in the body is the _____.

7. The normal state of the human body is called _____.

8. _____ occurs when the body is not working properly.

9. External environmental factors that affect the body include _____ and _____.

10. Viruses are external organisms carried through the air in _____.

11. Examples of viruses include _____, _____, and
    _____.

12. Illness, an accidental injury, a birth defect, or the normal sensory losses of aging may be the
    cause of a _____.

13. The Americans with Disabilities Act defines a person with a disability as someone who:

    a. _____

    b. _____

    c. _____

14. It takes longer for recovery in _____ adults because the growth rate of new
    cells _____.

15. An internal disorder that can happen at any age is an _____
    _____.

16. A person who normally functions well may have an emotional breakdown when
    _____ _____ becomes too great.

17. _____ is a normal response to illness.

18. Clients with mental illness need _____ and _____, just as
    clients with physical problems do.

19. Emotional and physical health are _____ on each other.

20. An emotional illness can cause a _____ illness.

21. Medications can cause _____ or _____.

22. The person who is ill experiences a _____ in physical and emotional energy,
    an _____ in physical discomfort, and perhaps chronic pain.

23. Roles in families _____ when a member is ill or has a disability.

24. The home health aide must be able to recognize, record, and report significant
    _____ and _____.

25. A change that can be observed or measured is called a _____.

26. List four signs of a physical change the aide should report to her supervisor.

    a. _____

    b. _____

    c. _____

    d. _____

27. Changes that cannot be observed but are experienced by the client are called
    _____.

28. Examples of symptoms are:

    a. _____

    b. _____

    c. _____

    d. _____

29. Signs obtained by the use of instruments are called _____ _____. They include _____, _____, _____ _____, and _____ _____.

30. _____ _____ must be measured accurately and regularly with changes reported to the _____.

31. The difference between the heat produced and the heat lost is the _____ _____ and is measured with a _____.

32. A person's body temperature varies throughout the day; it is _____ in the morning and _____ in the afternoon.

33. Name three factors that can raise a client's temperature.

    a. _____

    b. _____

    c. _____

34. Temperatures can be measured by _____, _____, or _____ using a digital thermometer.

35. A _____ or ear thermometer measures the temperature by inserting a probe into a person's ear.

36. When a client's body temperature is above normal, that is over _____ orally, the client is said to have a _____. Another term for fever is _____.

37. The temperature taken rectally is _____ _____ than the oral temperature.

38. An axillary temperature is _____ _____ than an oral temperature.

39. The _____ is the force of the blood pushing against the artery walls.

40. Pulse readings show the _____, _____, and volume of blood pulsing through the artery; _____ is the times per minute, _____ the evenness or regularity of the beat, _____ is the fullness of the beat.

41. The most common site for taking the pulse is the _____ artery.

42. Regularity when describing a pulse is described as _____ or _____.

43. An irregular pulse is one that indicates _____ heartbeats.

44. Volume of the pulse is described as _____, _____, or _____; if it is very weak, the term _____ is used.

45. The purpose of taking the pulse is to:

    a. _____

    b. _____

46. Pulse rate is described as the number of beats per _____.

47. Normal pulse rates are:

    a. _____ adults

    b. _____ children over 6 years of age

    c. _____ children under the age of 6

    d. _____ infants

48. A slow heartbeat is called _____ while a fast heartbeat is called _____.

49. _____ is the sum total of processes that exchange oxygen and carbon dioxide in the body; commonly known as _____.

50. Character of respirations is described as _____ or irregular; _____, difficult, _____, or deep; and _____ or quiet.

51. Terms used to describe respirations include: _____ difficult or labored breathing; _____ absence of breathing for a few moments; _____ bubbling sound heard when fluid or mucus gets caught in the air passages; _____ respirations that sound like snoring; and _____ respirations that are very rapid then stop and start again, often occurring before a client's death.

52. The normal respiratory rate for adults is _____ to _____ breaths per minute.

53. The amount of force the blood exerts against the walls of the arteries as it flows through them is called _____ _____.

54. Blood pressure is taken by the use of a _____ and a _____.

55. The higher number of the blood pressure reading is called _____; it represents the pressure when the heart is beating.

56. The lower number of the blood pressure reading is called _____; it represents the pressure when the heart is _____ between beats.

57. The _____ number is always recorded first and the _____ number last.

58. When a person has a blood pressure that is elevated above normal range, the person has _____; when it is below normal range the person has _____.

59. List five factors that can cause an increase in blood pressure.

    a. _____

    b. _____

    c. _____

    d. _____

    e. _____

60. In _____ _____ when a person changes position (like from sitting to standing), the person's blood pressure falls rapidly.

61. If your client has had a stroke or mastectomy, use the _____ arm only to take the blood pressure reading.

62. If the client has an IV or is receiving _____, you must take the blood pressure in the _____ _____.

63. Measure _____ with the client standing as straight as possible without his or her shoes on using a _____ _____ or a _____ against a wall.

64. Weight can be measured using a _____ _____ or for someone who cannot stand, using a _____ _____.

65. The normal state of awareness is called _____; a person is responsive and knows who and where they are.

66. Two temporary types of unconsciousness are _____ and _____; other types of unconsciousness are due to _____ _____ or _____.

67. List four levels of unconsciousness.

   a. _____

   b. _____

   c. _____

   d. _____

68. Two of the greatest potential problems for an unconscious client are _____ _____ and _____.

69. Exercises done to prevent contractures and loss of motion in the joints are called

   _____ _____ _____.

70. Two conditions that may occur when environmental conditions are extreme are _____ (heatstroke) and _____ (abnormally low internal body temperature under _____ °F).

71. List five signs and symptoms of hyperthermia.

   a. _____

   b. _____

   c. _____

   d. _____

   e. _____

72. Name three things you should do for a client you suspect has hyperthermia.

   a. _____

   b. _____

   c. _____

73. List five signs and symptoms of hypothermia.

   a. _____

   b. _____

   c. _____

   d. _____

   e. _____

74. To warm a person whom you suspect of having hypothermia, you should:

   a. _____

   b. _____

   c. _____

   d. _____

   e. _____

Matching. *Match each term with the correct definition.*

75. _____ bradycardia

76. _____ dyspnea

77. _____ apnea

78. _____ respiration

79. _____ rales

80. _____ Cheyne-Stokes respiration

81. _____ rhythm

a. the act of breathing

b. bubbling sound heard when fluid gets caught in the air passages

c. slow heartbeat

d. absence of breathing

e. difficult or labored breathing

f. evenness or regularity of the heartbeat

g. respirations that are very rapid, then stop, then start again

Multiple Choice. *Choose the correct answer or answers.*

82. Heredity can determine
   a. talents and abilities
   b. physical wellness
   c. height and weight
   d. all of these

83. The normal range of rectal temperature in an adult is
   a. 96.6°–98.6°F
   b. 99.6°–100.0°F
   c. 97.6°–99.6°F
   d. 94.6°–98.6°F

84. A client is febrile when his or her
   a. temperature is less than 96°F
   b. respiratory rate is below 16
   c. respiratory rate is above 24
   d. temperature is 100°F or above

85. This vital sign is measured using a watch with a second hand while feeling the artery pulsations in the wrist
   a. apical pulse
   b. brachial pulse
   c. respirations
   d. radial pulse

86. Normal respiratory rate in an adult is
   a. 16–20 breaths per minute
   b. 12–16 breaths per minute
   c. 8–16 breaths per minute
   d. 20–24 breaths per minute

87. A pulse that skips every fourth beat is called
   a. normal
   b. irregular
   c. faint
   d. bounding

88. Blood pressure is measured with a
    a. digital thermometer
    b. stethoscope
    c. sphygmomanometer
    d. doppler ultrasound

89. The first beat heard in the stethoscope when taking the blood pressure is referred to as the
    a. blood pressure
    b. diastolic
    c. systolic
    d. none of these

90. The last beat heard in the stethoscope when taking the blood pressure is referred to as the
    a. blood pressure
    b. diastolic
    c. systolic
    d. none of these

91. The normal pulse range of an infant is
    a. 100–140 beats per minute
    b. 80–120 beats per minute
    c. 70–110 beats per minute
    d. 60–100 beats per minute

Documentation Exercises. *Read the following descriptions and provide documentation for each scenario.*

92. You have checked the vital signs of your client. Temperature is 97.3°F, pulse is 86, respirations are 18, and blood pressure 126/88. Document these vital signs.

93. You assist your client who is ambulating with a walker. She walks 15 feet with dyspnea, then becomes so tired that she has to rest for five minutes. Document this.

94. Your client is spending most of her time in a wheelchair. You try to help her ambulate, but she tells you she prefers to remain in the wheelchair and watch television. You notice a reddened area on her right heel. After you have reported this to your supervisor, how would you document it?

Label the Diagram.

95. Refer to Figure 10–1. Label the sites where the pulse can be taken.

a._____

b._____

c._____

d. _____

e._____

f. _____

g._____

h. _____

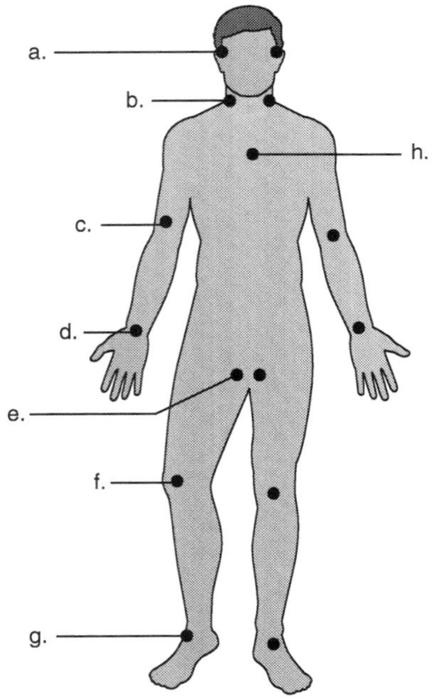

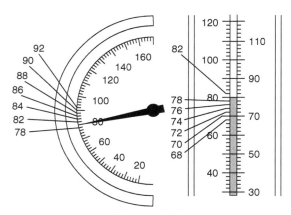

Figure 10–1

96. Refer to Figure 10–2. Take a reading at the closest line.

Figure 10–2

97. Refer to Figure 10–3. Determine the systolic and diastolic readings and write the number in the space provided.

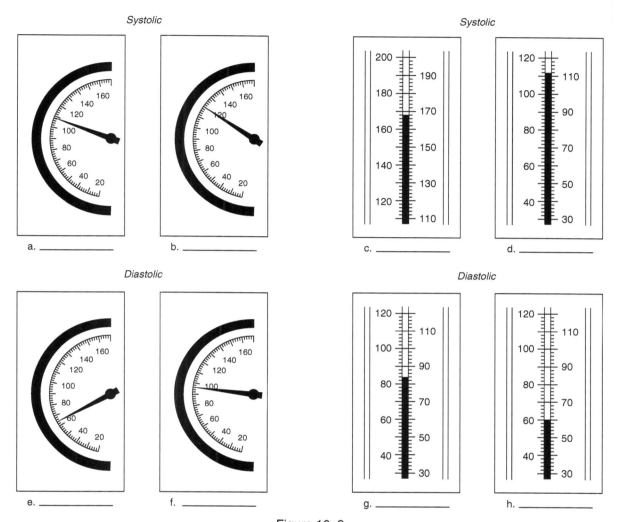

a. _____ b. _____ c. _____ d. _____

e. _____ f. _____ g. _____ h. _____

Figure 10–3

98. Read the following thermometers (Figure 10–4) and write the temperature in the space provided. Be sure to write "F" for Fahrenheit and "C" for Celsius.

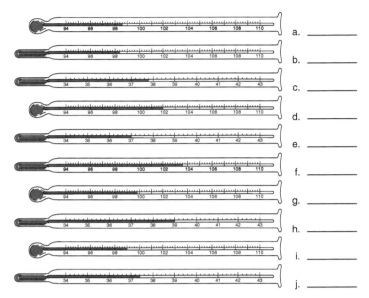

a. _____

b. _____

c. _____

d. _____

e. _____

f. _____

g. _____

h. _____

i. _____

j. _____

Figure 10–4

99. Read the following columns of mercury (Figure 10–5) and write the number in the space provided.

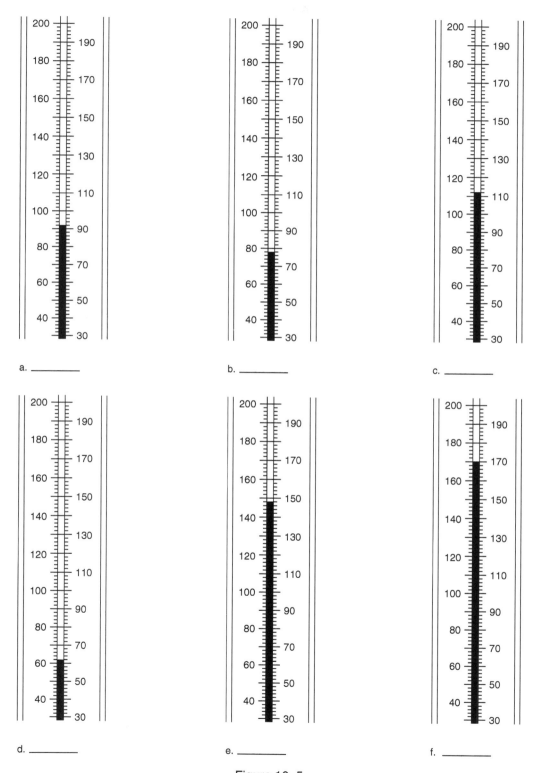

a. _____

b. _____

c. _____

d. _____

e. _____

f. _____

Figure 10–5

PRACTICE SITUATIONS

Case 1

You have been caring for Mrs. Moreno for several weeks. A nurse comes every week and sets up medications for the week. One of your responsibilities is to remind Mrs. Moreno to take her medications. When you arrive, you notice that she has not taken any medication all day. You remind her to take the medication. She tells you that God visited her and told her the medication is poisonous and not to take it. This is very unusual behavior for Mrs. Moreno.

Questions

1. What would you do?

2. Who would you call?

3. How will you convince Mrs. Moreno to take her medication?

Case 2

Your client, Mr. Pope, is usually very talkative. Today, however, he seems very quiet. His voice seems a little slurred. His face droops on the right side. You take his vital signs and discover his blood pressure is 210/100. You know this is very dangerous.

Questions

1. What do you do next?

2. How will you report his condition and at the same time keep him calm?

CROSSWORD PUZZLE

Across

1 restoring mental and physical abilities after an accident or illness

4 measurements of blood pressure, temperature, pulse, and respirations

6 difficult or labored respirations

8 begins suddenly and is usually severe

9 heartbeats per minute

12 those changes reported by the client

13 permanent shortening of muscle tissue causing deformity or distortion

17 respiration characterized by periods of apnea and periods of dyspnea

Down

2 slow pulse

3 absence of breathing

5 measurement of blood pressure when the heart is beating

7 bubbling sound from lungs when mucus or fluid is trapped in air passages

10 force exerted by blood on walls of blood vessels

11 a change that can be observed

14 one of the vital signs in which the breaths of a person are counted

15 lasts a long time

16 blood pressure measurement when heart is relaxing

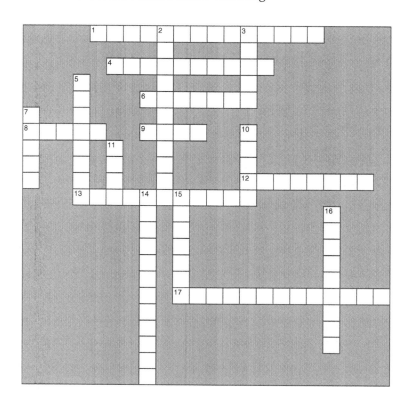

UNIT QUIZ

Read the scenario and answer the questions that follow.

Mr. Sanchez is a 45-year-old divorced male. He is successfully employed as a CPA for a large metropolitan business firm. He was married to a successful career woman for five years. They had no children.

During the last year of their marriage, Mr. Sanchez noticed he was having difficulty walking at times for no apparent reason. He ignored this for awhile, but associates at work strongly urged him to see his health care provider. Mr. Sanchez did this, and after a series of extensive tests, he was diagnosed with multiple sclerosis.

Mrs. Sanchez, who could not cope with this news, sought a divorce. Mr. Sanchez was devastated, but through the help of family and friends came through this ordeal. Six months passed and more generalized weakness and fatigue occurred, followed by a severe urinary tract infection. Recovery was slow and Mr. Sanchez's place of employment was having difficulty justifying his increased absences and decreased amount of work productivity. After six more months Mr. Sanchez was released from work on a permanent disability.

Mr. Sanchez found it more and more difficult with ADLs—showering, eating, getting to the store, and generally caring for himself. Mr. Sanchez fell at home and fractured both hips. After his hospitalization, the social worker at the hospital before his discharge arranged for home care services. Mr. Sanchez also suffered from severe depression.

Short Answer/Fill in the Blanks. *Complete the following sentences with the correct word or words.*

1. A change that can be observed or measured is called a _____.

2. Changes that cannot be observed but are experienced by the client are called

   _____.

3. Signs of multiple sclerosis discussed in the above scenario are:

   a. _____

   b. _____

4. Symptoms of multiple sclerosis experienced by Mr. S. are:

   a. _____

   b. _____

5. Signs obtained by the use of an instrument are called _____

   _____.

6. A vital sign you would check when Mr. S. complains of symptoms of urinary tract infection would be his _____.

7. Mr. S. was diagnosed with depression. List three stressors that he experienced.

   a. _____

   b. _____

   c. _____

8. A person who has a physical or mental disability that substantially limits one or more major life activities has a _____.

9. The _____ _____ _____ _____
   is a national law protecting the rights of people with disabilities.

10. After an aide has seen the normal reactions of the client, deviations or changes that could be serious can be recognized and should be reported to the _____.

11. The vital signs abbreviated as T, P, R, B/P are: _____, _____, _____, and _____ _____.

12. List the average temperature ranges.

    oral: _____, axillary: _____, and rectal: _____.

13. You check Mr. S.'s pulse and obtain a reading of 56. This is called _____. His usual rate is between 68 to 82. What should you do with this reading?

14. Orthostatic hypotension would be detected in Mr. S. by checking his blood pressure _____ and _____.

15. Mr. S.'s normal respiratory rate should be between _____ to _____.

Matching. *Match each term with the correct definition.*

16. _____ apical
17. _____ apical-radial pulse
18. _____ brachial
19. _____ coma
20. _____ dyspnea
21. _____ exhalation
22. _____ hypertension
23. _____ hyperthermia
24. _____ hypothermia
25. _____ inhalation
26. _____ rales
27. _____ respiration
28. _____ somnolence
29. _____ stupor
30. _____ tachycardia

a. blood pressure reading above 160/90

b. heart rate above 100

c. temperature below 96

d. inward intake of breath

e. exchange of oxygen and carbon dioxide

f. bubbling sound when fluid gets trapped in the lungs

g. outward breath

h. artery located in bend of arm

i. pulse located at heart

j. done to check to see if radial pulse is the same as apical pulse

k. difficult or labored breathing

l. heatstroke

m. client can answer questions, is confused, fades in and out of sleep

n. client is restless, only aroused by continuous stimulation

o. responds only to painful stimuli, if at all

Multiple Choice. *Choose the correct answer or answers.*

31. Equipment needed to take an apical pulse includes

    a. stethoscope

    b. watch with second hand

    c. alcohol pads

    d. all of the above

32. After gathering equipment, the next step in taking an apical pulse is

    a. listen carefully for the heartbeat

    b. place stethoscope in ears

    c. tell client what you plan to do

    d. clean stethoscope diaphragm and earpieces with alcohol

33. After obtaining the apical pulse and removing stethoscope from client's chest, you should

    a. record reading in notes

    b. clean stethoscope diaphragm and earpieces with alcohol

    c. report abnormal results to nurse

    d. all of the above

34. When using a tympanic thermometer, you should

    a. Apply a clean disposable probe on the thermometer.

    b. In an adult, pull top of ear up and back and gently insert probe into ear.

    c. In an adult, pull earlobe down and back and gently insert probe into ear.

    d. Shake the thermometer to get the mercury to go down after use.

35. When taking an oral temperature with a digital thermometer, you need to

    a. First turn the thermometer on and insert under the axilla. Wait for beep to stop, about 10 to 20 seconds. Record temperature.

    b. Apply sheath cover to end of thermometer. Place probe tip well under the tongue in sublingual pocket. Tell client to close mouth, turn thermometer on and wait for beep to stop, about 10 to 20 seconds. Record temperature.

    c. Turn thermometer on. Apply sheath cover to end of thermometer, place probe tip on top of the tongue. Tell client to close mouth, and wait for beep to stop, about 10 to 20 seconds. Record temperature.

    d. Wash hands and apply gloves. Apply sheath cover to end of thermometer. Place probe tip well under tongue in sublingual pocket. Tell client to close mouth, turn thermometer on and wait for beep to stop, about 10 to 20 seconds. Remove plastic probe cover and discard in wastebasket. Turn thermometer off. Record temperature. Remove gloves and wash hands.

36. Counting respirations involves

    a. Counting after the pulse is taken so the client is not aware that you are counting respirations.

    b. One rise and fall of the chest counts as one respiration. Count the number of respirations during a full 1-minute period.

    c. Observing how deeply the client breathes, regularity of the rhythm pattern, and sound of breathing. Report changes or difficulty breathing to the nurse.

    d. All of the above are correct.

37. How high should you inflate the blood pressure cuff beyond the point at which you last felt the pulse?

    a. 10 mm HG

    b. 20 mm HG

    c. 30 mm HG

    d. 40 mm HG

38. You arrive at Mrs. Jones's home in the winter to discover the heat is off. Mrs. Jones is shivering slightly, complains of pains in her hands, and is slowly moving about the room. Checking her vital signs: pulse is 60 and weak, blood pressure is 86/60, temperature is 95°F. You suspect that she has

    a. hypothermia

    b. Alzheimer's disease

    c. hyperthermia

    d. hypothyroidism

39. Things you can do to help Mrs. Jones include

    a. Wrap her in a warm blanket, quilt, towels, or extra clothes.

    b. Use a hot bottle or electric heating pad on her abdomen.

    c. Give her a warm drink or small quantities of warm (not hot) food.

    d. Call 911 and notify the case manager.

    e. All of the above are correct.

40. Meeting the special needs of the unconscious client includes

    a. Performing mouth care every 2 hours and when the client vomits.

    b. Repositioning every 2 hours to prevent pressure sores from forming.

    c. Every 2 hours, checking perineal area and bed linens to see if they are dry.

    d. Wiping eyes clean in A.M. and P.M. Use Artificial Tears.

    e. All of the above are correct.

UNIT 11   MENTAL HEALTH

LEARNING OBJECTIVES

After studying this unit, you should be able to:

■ Identify several common emotions

■ Identify how a physical response can result from an emotional reaction

■ Discuss the tasks of personality development defined by Erikson

■ Define mental illness

■ Define psychology, stress, mental health, and adjustments

■ Differentiate between external and internal stimuli

■ Identify the major signs of depression

TERMS TO DEFINE

■ adjustment

■ anxiety disorder

■ bipolar disorder

■ cognitive

■ compulsion

■ delusion

■ depression

■ emotions

■ external stimulus

■ hallucinations

■ internal stimulus

■ mental disorder

■ obsession

■ optimist

■ pessimist

■ post-traumatic stress disorder

■ psychology

■ psychosis

■ schizophrenia

■ stress

APPLICATION EXERCISES

Short Answer/Fill in the Blanks. *Complete the following sentences with the correct word or words.*

1. The science of human behavior is called _____.

2. An adjustment is the _____ a person makes in behavior to cope with a situation.

3. _____ _____ cause automatic or unconscious reactions within the body while _____ _____ come from outside the body and bring conscious reaction.

4. A strong, generalized feeling is called an _____ and is neither good nor bad.

5. The well-adjusted individual has a good _____ and can be _____ in new or difficult situations.

6. The body's communication center is the _____.

7. People who are depressed show signs of feeling extremely _____.

8. The stages in the development of one's _____ are determined over an individual's lifespan.

9. According to Erikson, _____ and _____ influences are significant during the _____ and _____ phase of the individual.

10. The personality task to be mastered for a middle-aged adult focuses on _____ versus _____.

11. An _____ feels more pleasant emotions and has a brighter outlook on life.

12. A _____ has a differing viewpoint and tends to take a negative view of situations.

13. Mentally healthy people learn to make their _____ work for them.

14. Clients who are often frightened and worried about their health, may have strong outbursts, and become _____. A home health aide must not only deal with his or her own emotional needs, but must think of the _____ _____ _____.

15. _____ is defined as a mentally or physically disruptive influence or upsetting condition.

16. Stress may be seen as _____, depression, silence, _____, crying, _____, jealousy, and _____.

17. Examples of possible stressors when a family member is ill are:

    a. _____

    b. _____.

    c. _____

18. A person is said to have a _____ _____ if she or he is having difficulty functioning satisfactorily in society as a result of changes in thoughts, behavior, personality, or emotion.

19. Individuals with _____ _____ live a fairly normal life but are always worrying. This disorder causes the person to be very tense, _____, and affects the person's ability to sleep; _____ _____ are quite common.

20. _____ _____ _____ _____ develops after terrifying events, seen often in soldiers returning home from war or rape victims.

21. _____ are thoughts, images, or ideas that repeatedly go through a person's mind while _____ are acts that correspond with these obsessions.

22. A person with _____ _____ can alternate from being excessively depressed to very elated and back again, with little reason for these mood swings.

23. Depressed persons have difficulty paying _____ and may also be _____.

24. Three negative thoughts caused by depression are:

    a. _____

    b. _____

    c. _____

25. Three physical changes caused by depression are:

    a. _____

    b. _____

    c. _____

26. Depressed people are _____ to control the way they feel.

27. The home health aide is in a unique position to recognize changes in the client that could indicate signs of _____ thoughts.

28. If the home health aide notices signs that indicate the client is having suicidal thoughts, the aide needs to _____ _____ _____.

29. A serious condition in which the thinking process is distorted by hallucinations, delusions, or both is called _____.

30. Common signs and symptoms of _____ are disorganized thoughts, bizarre behaviors, attention deficits, and withdrawal with common delusions involving themes of grandeur, persecution, or religion.

Matching. *Match the tasks of personality development with the age.*

31. _____ establish intimate personal relationships with mate.

32. _____ recognize oneself as independent from mother

33. _____ review life events and examine how they influenced development

34. _____ demonstrate physical and mental skills ability

35. _____ learn to trust

36. _____ recognize oneself as a family member

37. _____ develop a sense of individuality as a sexual human being

38. _____ live a satisfying and productive life

a. birth to 18 months

b. 18 months to 3 years

c. 3–6 years

d. 6–12 years

e. 12–20 years

f. 20–35 years

g. 35–59 years

h. 50 plus

Multiple Choice. *Choose the correct answer or answers.*

39. A client's illness

    a. can cause temporary emotional changes in the client's personality

    b. generally has no effect on the client's personality

    c. can affect the home health aide

    d. none of these

40. The home health aide caring for an emotionally upset client needs to

    a. feel free to have strong outbursts of anger at the client, if they are justified

    b. be able to cope with his or her own emotional needs

    c. be kind and understanding with the emotionally upset client

    d. b and c only

41. Delirium, depression, and anxiety disorders are examples of

    a. strange ways of thinking

    b. mental disorders

    c. emotions

    d. behavior seen in persons with character disorders

42. A home health aide caring for a depressed client should

    a. perform all necessary tasks for the client

    b. never leave the client alone

    c. encourage the client to use his or her remaining capabilities

43. When illness strikes a family, it can cause

    a. anxiety   c. financial loss

    b. worry   d. all of these

44. When a client seems to be very apathetic about his or her plan of care, you should

    a. assume he or she is ill   c. notify your case manager

    b. forget about it   d. tell a family member

45. Ways home health aides can help the client with mental health issues include

    a. being aware of the client's mental health status

    b. reporting all statements of self-harm or suicide to the nurse or case manager

    c. respond to clients in a supportive and nonjudgmental way

    d. all of the above

Documentation Exercises. *Read the following descriptions and provide documentation for each scenario.*

46. You are caring for a 78-year-old lady who recently had cataract surgery. She tells you that she sees a beautiful pink lake with blue fishes swimming all around. How would you document this?

47. You arrive at your client's home. He is sitting in the closet. He tells you to be very quiet because the Germans have landed on the roof. If you make too much noise, they will come down and arrest you. How would you document this?

48. You are caring for a 50-year-old lady whose husband has recently died. You find her staring out the window in her bedroom. She is weeping and tells you there is no point in going on. There is no one who cares for her any longer. Document this.

PRACTICE SITUATIONS

Case 1

You are caring for a client who is very depressed. Usually, she sits quietly looking out the window all day without talking. She will answer questions only with short answers. Today, when you arrive, Mrs. Jose is talking loudly, smiling, and seems very glad to see you.

Questions

1. What do you think has happened?
2. Do you need to report this?

Case 2

You are caring for Mr. Fife. He has a psychiatric diagnosis. He cannot care for his needs. You are to give him a bath, change his clothes, and prepare food for two meals. You are concerned about his careless smoking habits. He drops lighted matches on the floor. Sometimes, he will have as many as three cigarettes going at one time.

Questions

1. What can you do to prevent a fire?
2. Do you need to report this behavior to anyone?
3. Is there someone who can advise you?

CROSSWORD PUZZLE

Across

3 change a person makes in behavior to deal with a situation
5 hearing voices, seeing bugs, or other things
9 science of human behavior
11 person who usually has a positive disposition
12 person who usually has a negative view of situations

Down

1 serious condition in which the thought process is distorted by hallucinations, delusions, or both
2 false beliefs
4 difficulty functioning in society as a result of changes in thoughts, behavior, personality, or emotions
6 acts that correspond with obsessions
7 serious disorder where persons are extremely sad, feel worthless, helpless, and express feelings of guilt
8 strong, generalized feelings
10 pertaining to the mental process of thought, including perception, reasoning, intuition, and memory

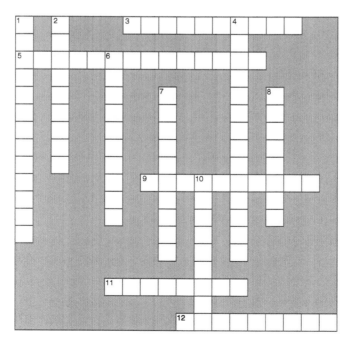

UNIT QUIZ

Short Answer/Fill in the Blanks. *Complete the following sentences with the correct word or words.*

1. The study of the way the mind works and how emotions and feelings affect human behavior is called _____.

2. The _____ acts as the body's communication center.

3. In some conditions, chemical imbalances within the body or brain and nerve cell damage can cause _____ _____ _____.

4. _____ may cause physical reactions, trigger release of hormones, and produce unusual results.

5. Disposition is the usual mood of an individual and includes _____ and _____.

6. Temporary changes in personality may be caused by _____.

7. _____ is the change a person makes in behavior to deal with a situation.

8. Three examples of anxiety disorders are:

    a. _____

    b. _____

    c. _____

9. Two ways of strengthening the body's resistance to stress include:

    a. _____

    b. _____

10. The most common treatments today for mental disorders are:

    a. _____

    b. _____

True or False. *Answer the following statements true (T) or false (F).*

11. T   F   Mood disorders are the most common mental disorders for people of all ages.

12. T   F   Defense mechanisms, such as withdrawal and anger, are harmful to the client who uses these all the time.

13. T   F   People with physical disabilities may display periods of hopelessness.

14. T   F   People with mental illness are not really ill.

15. T   F   You may not always be able to meet all the needs of the client with mental illness.

16. T   F   It is important for you as a homemaker/home health aide to present a positive attitude toward the client and the family.

17. T   F   Emotions are common to all people and are labeled as either good or bad.

18. T   F   Symptoms of panic attacks include shortness of breath, pounding heart and lightheadedness, and people may think they are having a heart attack.

19. T   F   Compulsions are thoughts, images, or ideas that are repeated over and over again in a person's mind.

20. T   F   Mentally healthy people learn to make their emotions work for them.

Matching. *Match each term with the proper definition.*

21. _____ internal stimuli
22. _____ external stimuli
23. _____ emotion
24. _____ mental disorder
25. _____ hallucinations
26. _____ delirium
27. _____ depression
28. _____ psychosis
29. _____ delusions
30. _____ obsessions

a. serious condition in which the thinking process is distorted by hallucination or delusions

b. disturbance of consciousness, making it difficult for a person to focus or shift attention

c. ranges from emotional "blue feeling" to serious condition with client unable to function outside home

d. a strong, generalized feeling

e. cause automatic or unconscious reactions within the body

f. difficulty functioning in society as a result of changes in thoughts, behavior, or emotions

g. outside the body stimuli

h. hearing voices, seeing bugs, or other things

i. false beliefs

j. thoughts, images, or ideas that repeatedly go through a person's mind

Multiple Choice. *Choose the correct answer or answers.*

31. During your visits, Mrs. Heller complains you don't dust right or fold the laundry properly. After you clean her floor, she inspects it for shine. Despite her arthritis, you have seen her refold towels you just put away. Her need for perfection has made the aides very tense when caring for her. You realize she has signs of

    a. schizophrenia
    b. obsessive-compulsive disorder
    c. depression
    d. bipolar disorder

32. Miss Anderson was a nurse in her 20s and 30s but now is confined to her home due to mental health problems. Some visits will find her sitting in a chair rocking throughout your two-hour visit. Other times, she is talking to herself, peering behind curtains, and whispering that the neighbors are beaming radiation waves into her home. Miss Anderson has

    a. schizophrenia
    b. obsessive-compulsive disorder
    c. depression
    d. bipolar disorder

33. Mr. Arthur is a retired car salesman. He is sometimes found in his living room looking at car magazines, talking about all the latest car models, and boasting how he was asked to show the new employees how to sell cars. Other times, he is quiet and withdrawn, won't leave his bed so you can change the linens, and tells you to go away. His actions indicate signs of

    a. schizophrenia
    b. obsessive-compulsive disorder
    c. depression
    d. bipolar disorder

34. You are assigned to help care for Mrs. Wall, her newborn twins, and a 3-year-old son. Mrs. Wall was initially very upbeat about her new family, but recently she talks about how stressful it is caring for them all and that she feels tired and overwhelmed. She won't eat the lunches you prepare and spends little time with the twins. Her conversations usually end with her crying. She has signs of postpartum

    a. schizophrenia   c. depression

    b. obsessive-compulsive disorder   d. bipolar disorder

35. Mr. Katz has been battling depression since having a stroke. Off and on he tells you the end might be near, but by the end of your visits, he is joking and laughing. Today, he confides in you that he has been saving up his pills for the "big day." You need to

    a. Call the local Psych Crisis Center.

    b. Notify his health care provider.

    c. Tell your case manager immediately about this report.

    d. Do nothing as it's not your responsibility.

36. The home health aide needs to be aware of stressors when dealing with home health care clients and should

    a. identify healthy ways to relieve everyday stress

    b. know that it's alright to occasionally yell at a client

    c. inform the case manager when clients' demands are causing personal conflict

    d. all of the above

SECTION 5
Body Systems and Common Disorders

UNIT 12   DIGESTION AND NUTRITION

LEARNING OBJECTIVES

After studying this unit, you should be able to:

■ List the organs of the digestive system and their function

■ Discuss common disorders of the digestive system

■ Explain the purpose and use of the food guide pyramid

■ List four guidelines for planning menus for the client

■ Name six guidelines for purchasing food

■ Describe five guidelines for preparing food

■ Identify common food allergies

■ List at least seven special diets and foods allowed on each diet

■ List medical conditions that the above diets would be used for

■ Explain care for clients with various types of feeding tubes

■ Demonstrate the following:
Procedure 19   Feeding the Client

TERMS TO DEFINE

■ aspirate
■ bland diet
■ calorie-controlled diet
■ clear liquid diet
■ convenience foods
■ delicatess
■ diabetic diet
■ diuretic
■ emesis
■ empty calorie
■ enzymes
■ fiber
■ food allergy
■ food guide pyramid

■ full-liquid diet
■ gastrostomy
■ hiatal hernia
■ high-fiber diet
■ low-sodium diet
■ lactose
■ malnutrition
■ Meals on Wheels
■ metabolism
■ nutrition
■ perishable
■ peristalsis
■ pureed diet
■ reflux

- soft diet
- total parenteral nutrition (TPN)
- ulcer
- vegetarians

APPLICATION EXERCISES

Short Answer/Fill in the Blanks. *Complete the following sentences with the correct word or words.*

1. The sum of a combination of processes by which the body receives and uses food and nutrients is called _____.

2. Those parts of food that cannot be used by the body are expelled as _____ or _____.

3. In the body, the fuel is _____; the process of burning this fuel is called _____.

4. Digestion begins in the _____. In the saliva, chemical substances called _____ start breaking down starchy foods into food products used by the rest of the body.

5. Food is moved through the esophagus and the stomach by the process of _____.

6. Bile enters the small intestine and breaks up _____ so that they can be absorbed.

7. Vomiting or _____ is caused by the voluntary and involuntary muscles forcing food backward through the mouth.

8. An elastic, muscular organ that holds the food and secretes and mixes it in gastric juices is called the _____.

9. The small intestine consists of the _____, _____, and _____.

10. A backflow of digestive juices into the lower portion of the esophagus, causing irritation to the lining is called _____.

11. _____ occur when there is a break in the protective mucous membrane of the stomach or first part of the intestine.

12. Three tips to prevent reflux are:

    a. _____

    b. _____

    c. _____

13. The professional person who evaluates the client's medical needs and prepares the meal plan is called a _____.

14. Indicate in the list below the percentage of each food group recommended in a balanced diet.

    a. _____ fat   c. _____ simple sugars

    b. _____ protein   d. _____ carbohydrates

15. A guide to healthful daily food choices is the _____ _____ _____.

16. Dietary guidelines for Americans include:

    a. _____

    b. _____

    c. _____

    d. _____

    e. _____

17. Many women and adolescent girls need to eat more _____
    _____ foods to get the calcium they need for healthy bones throughout life.

18. Vitamin and mineral supplements taken regularly in large amounts above 100% of
    recommended daily dose can be _____.

19. Iron supplements are often recommended for _____ and some menstruating
    women.

20. Research has shown that mothers who had babies born with birth defects and Down
    syndrome had low levels of _____ _____, so a supplement is
    now recommended.

21. Since 1990, all packaged and processed foods carry a _____
    _____ with nutritional information to help you plan a balanced diet. Because
    many people are on a salt-restricted diet, the food industry has to list the amount of
    _____ in food on this label.

22. List what counts as one serving for the following food group items.

    a. _____ milk   f. _____ fish, poultry, meat

    b. _____ cheese   g. _____ peanut butter

    c. _____ leafy vegetables h. _____ bread

    d. _____ cooked vegetables i. _____ cereal, rice, or pasta

    e. _____ egg   j. _____ fruit

23. The main sources of saturated fat are _____ _____ and
    tropical oils.

24. List five recommendations for reducing fat and cholesterol in the American diet.

    a. _____

    b. _____

    c. _____

    d. _____

    e. _____

25. Commonly called junk foods, _____ _____ foods are high in
    sugars and fats and low in proteins, minerals, and vitamins.

26. Signs a person is well nourished include _____ hair, _____
    skin, good posture, and _____ flesh.

27. _____ is poor nourishment, which most often occurs when the body does not
    get a full, balanced diet.

28. Early signs of malnutrition are _____ _____ and a constant feeling of _____.

29. As the malnutrition progresses, the symptoms become more severe and include _____ abdomen, a dull film over the _____, hair that is _____ and _____, and bones that become _____.

30. It is generally recommended that a person drink _____ to _____ glasses of water per day.

31. Three reasons to include ample water in the diet are:

    a. _____

    b. _____

    c. _____

32. The home health aide needs to consider the general guidelines for good nutrition when preparing meals for the client, and also consider the client's _____ _____.

33. A service that brings hot meals to homebound persons is called _____ _____ _____.

34. A food allergy is any negative reaction to a food that involves the _____ _____.

35. List five factors to consider when planning a meal for your client.

    a. _____

    b. _____

    c. _____

    d. _____

    e. _____

36. Five practical guidelines for shopping are:

    a. _____

    b. _____

    c. _____

    d. _____

    e. _____

37. Three foods a client on a low-calorie diet should avoid are:

    a. _____

    b. _____

    c. _____

38. A drug called a _____ is given to people with high blood pressure and causes _____ to be flushed from the body, causing muscle cramps and muscular weakness.

39. The diet prescribed for clients with difficulties in swallowing is called a _____ diet.

40. If it is necessary to feed a client, the food will be digested better in a _____ position.

41. Clients who tend to choke easily will choke less if the liquid is _____ .

42. Clients who cannot swallow are sometimes fed through a _____ tube.

43. For clients who cannot be nourished by being fed through the mouth or gastrostomy tube, they may receive intravenous nutrition called _____ _____ _____ (TPN).

44. Three foods excluded from a soft diet are:

    a. _____

    b. _____

    c. _____

45. Four foods included in a diabetic diet are:

    a. _____

    b. _____

    c. _____

    d. _____

46. Three foods excluded from a low-sodium diet are:

    a. _____

    b. _____

    c. _____

47. Three foods you could prepare on a low-fat diet are:

    a. _____

    b. _____

    c. _____

48. Three foods excluded from a diabetic diet are:

    a. _____

    b. _____

    c. _____

49. List three foods you could prepare on a full-liquid diet.

    a. _____

    b. _____

    c. _____

50. Three foods included on a high-fiber diet are:

    a. _____

    b. _____

    c. _____

51. List four foods that are high in potassium.

    a. _____

    b. _____

    c. _____

    d. _____

52. Three functions of vitamin C are:

    a. _____

    b. _____

    c. _____

53. List three sources of vitamin C.

    a. _____

    b. _____

    c. _____

Matching. *Match each term with the correct definition.*

54. _____ carbohydrates

55. _____ proteins

56. _____ fats

57. _____ minerals

58. _____ water

59. _____ calorie

60. _____ metabolism

61. _____ vitamins

a. a tasteless, odorless liquid

b. measure of heat produced by the body when using a specific portion of food

c. organic substances vital to certain metabolic functions and needed to prevent deficiency

d. sum total of processes needed for the breakdown of food and absorption of nutrients

e. sugars or starches that are made up of carbon, hydrogen, and oxygen and deliver quick energy to the body

f. inorganic elements essential in tissue building and in regulation of body fluids

g. compounds composed of amino acids needed for growth and tissue repair

h. oily substances made up of glycerin and fatty acids

True or False. *Answer the following statements true (T) or false (F).*

62. T F The average individual should walk 30 minutes a day.

63. T F It is important to eat foods from each of the five major food groups each day.

64. T F It is acceptable to eat candy and sweet desserts as long as a person is not overweight.

65. T F The normal person requires 40 nutrients for good health.

66. T F   If you take vitamin supplements, you can eat whatever you want.

67. T F   Whole grain bread and cereals are good sources of fiber.

68. T F   Milk is a good source of calcium and iron.

69. T F   Women and adolescent girls need to eat more calcium-rich foods.

70. T F   Pregnant women generally need an iron supplement.

71. T F   Most health authorities recommend a diet low in fat and cholesterol.

72. T F   The risk of heart disease increases in persons who have high cholesterol blood levels, have high blood pressure, and smoke.

73. T F   Animal fats are not the source of saturated fats in most diets.

74. T F   To lower cholesterol, you need to eat less animal fat, use oils and fats sparingly, use small amounts of salad dressings, and use skim or low-fat dairy products.

75. T F   Empty-calorie foods are foods with no calories.

76. T F   Calories that are not used by the body are turned into fat for storage.

Multiple Choice. *Choose the correct answer or answers.*

77. Daily food guides recommend

   a. 4–5 servings of meat daily

   b. 2–3 servings of breads daily

   c. 2–3 servings of dairy products daily

   d. 4–5 servings of fats daily

78. The foods highest in vitamin C are

   a. fish, beef, and tuna

   b. citrus fruits, melons, broccoli

   c. cheese, milk, and yogurt

   d. rice, pasta, bread

79. Vitamin B$_{12}$ is essential for

   a. metabolism

   b. health red blood cells

   c. treatment of pernicious anemia

   d. all of these

80. Vitamin K is essential for

   a. growth

   b. normal clotting of blood

   c. shiny hair and teeth

   d. none of these

81. Good sources of vitamin D include

   a. spinach

   b. margarine, butter

   c. sunshine, milk

   d. dark green leafy vegetables

82. Low-sodium diets are usually prescribed for

   a. headaches

   b. diabetes

   c. intestinal problems

   d. heart disease, fluid retention

83. Good sources of calcium are

   a. milk and milk products

   b. red meat and fish

   c. green leafy vegetables

   d. breads and rice

Documentation Exercises. *Read the following descriptions and provide documentation for each scenario.*

84. You prepare a meal for your client. He picks at the food and eats only a few bites of the potatoes, a small bite of the meat, and none of the carrots or salad. How would you document his appetite?

85. Your client has been placed on a high-potassium diet. What would you serve him and how would you document it?

Label the Diagram

86. Label the sections of the food pyramid with the types of food and number of recommended servings; refer to Figure 12–1.

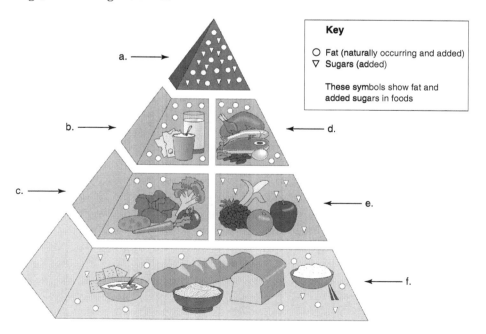

Figure 12–1

a. _____   d. _____

b. _____   e. _____

c. _____   f. _____

87. Label the parts of the digestive system on the diagram; refer to Figure 12–2.

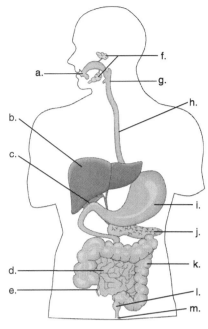

a. _____

b. _____

c. _____

d. _____

e. _____

f. _____

g. _____

h. _____

i. _____

j. _____

k. _____

l. _____

m. _____

Figure 12–2

PRACTICE SITUATIONS

Case 1

The client you are caring for is on a special diet. She is very fussy about her food. You have asked her to tell you what she would like to have you prepare for her lunch. You have prepared what she asked for. When you put the plate in front of her, she looks at you in disgust and states that you have not prepared what she asked for. You are very upset about this behavior. In fact, you are ready to grab your coat and leave.

Questions

1. What other alternatives are there?

2. Can you think of another solution?

3. Can you think of any reason she would behave this way?

Case 2

You are caring for Mr. Talimentes, who is very malnourished. His wife died several months ago. They were very close, and he has lost 30 pounds since she died. Your task is to prepare a high-calorie meal for him.

Questions

1. What can you do to encourage him to eat?

2. Can you think of ways to make his food higher in calories?

CROSSWORD PUZZLE

Across

2 salt-restricted diet

5 digestive juices

9 vomiting

14 IV therapy when one cannot eat or have gastrostomy tube

Down

1 negative reaction to a food

3 person who has problems with insulin production

4 poor nourishment

6 tube in stomach for feedings

7 process by which the body receives and uses food

8 diet of semisolid foods, foods put in blender

10 service that brings hot foods to the homebound

11 break in the mucous membrane of the stomach

12 meatless diet

13 bulk-forming foods, bran

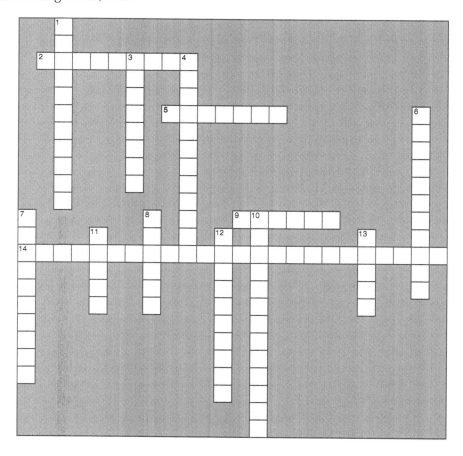

UNIT QUIZ

Short Answer/Fill in the Blanks. *Complete the following sentences with the correct word or words.*

1. The body needs food for _____, _____ _____, comfort, and satiety.

2. Digestion begins when food enters the _____.

3. A _____ diet generally does not contain animal products.

4. The member of the health care team in hospitals and nursing homes who evaluates diet needs, recommends sound diet plans, and educates clients regarding healthy diets is a _____.

5. To have a nutritious diet, people must eat a _____ of foods.

6. Poor nourishment is called _____ and most often occurs when the body does not get a full, balanced diet.

7. The nutrient that flushes out food wastes and helps to prevent constipation and cancer of the colon is _____.

8. Three ways to decrease salt in the diet include:

    a. _____

    b. _____

    c. _____

9. _____ _____ occurs when the upper part of the stomach protrudes through the esophageal opening of the diaphragm into the lung cavity.

10. List two examples of foods in each of these food groups.

    a. Breads and cereals: _____ _____

    b. Milk and cheese: _____ _____

    c. Vegetables: _____ _____

    d. Fruits: _____ _____

    e. Meats and poultry: _____ _____

    f. Fats, oils, sweets: _____ _____

Matching. *Match each term with the correct definition.*

11. _____   aspirate
12. _____   carbohydrates
13. _____   emesis
14. _____   enzymes
15. _____   food
16. _____   gastrostomy
17. _____   metabolism
18. _____   peristalsis
19. _____   proteins

a. inhaling food and foreign materials into lungs

b. feeding tube inserted into stomach

c. vomiting of food, bile, and stomach acids

d. wavelike muscle action that moves food through digestive tract

e. process of burning body fuel

f. fuel burned by digestive system to provide body energy

g. chemical substances that break down food

h. sugars or starches that give quick energy to the body

i. compounds composed of amino acids needed for growth and tissue repair

Multiple Choice. *Choose the correct answer or answers.*

20. Good nutrition is needed for
   a. proper growth and development
   b. healing of wounds
   c. maintaining proper body functions
   d. all of these

21. For bone and teeth formation, people need
   a. calcium and phosphorus
   b. iron
   c. sodium
   d. none of these

22. A general diet means that
   a. there are no dieting restrictions
   b. only certain meats are allowed
   c. a great amount of fluid must be taken with each meal
   d. the client will receive high-protein snacks

23. Clients with chewing difficulties should have
   a. a full-liquid diet
   b. a high-potassium diet
   c. a bland diet
   d. a soft diet

24. A client who is on low-salt diet asks you to stop at a fast-food restaurant before you come the next time and bring a large order of french fries. You should
   a. bring the food as requested
   b. substitute fried onion rings for the french fries
   c. remind the client that french fires are restricted, but you will talk to the case manager
   d. tell the client that this behavior has to stop

25. When you are planning meals for a client, you should remember
    a. that combining textures makes meals more appealing
    b. to prepare foods that vary in color
    c. to use a lot of herbs and spices
    d. none of these

26. Before eating, the client should be allowed to
    a. perform oral hygiene   c. wash his or her hands
    b. urinate   d. all of these

27. Causes of dehydration include all of the following except
    a. vomiting   c. diarrhea
    b. excessive fluid intake   d. excessive sweating

28. When feeding a client, you should offer food
    a. as the client prefers
    b. in a clockwise fashion
    c. as you would eat the food, one item at a time

29. Eating and drinking aids for clients with disabilities may include
    a. feeding cup   c. cutlery with built-up handles
    b. food bumper or plate with curved edge   d. all of the above

30. John has a peanut allergy. He needs to read labels and avoid
    a. peanut cooking oil   c. cookies and cakes made with peanuts
    b. walnuts and pecans   d. peanut butter

31. Mr. Walters is on dialysis and follows a renal low-potassium diet. Foods to avoid serving are
    a. orange juice   c. milk and cheese
    b. baked potato   d. green leafy vegetables

32. Pregnant women should include the following foods in their diet
    a. milk and cheese   c. dry beans and whole grain breads
    b. green leafy vegetables   d. lean meats

33. Foods to avoid on a diabetic diet include
    a. tomatoes and salads   c. soda and fruit juices
    b. canned fruits in heavy syrup d. jello

34. Vitamin D is essential for
    a. growth of bones   c. regulating calcium and phosphorus
    b. health of eyes   d. carbohydrate metabolism

35. Best sources of vitamin D are
    a. dried beans and fortified cereals   c. sunshine
    b. egg yolk   d. fortified milk

36. Vitamin K is essential for
    a. growth of bones
    b. prevention of pellagra
    c. metabolism of proteins
    d. normal clotting of blood

37. Sources of vitamin K include
    a. spinach
    b. cabbage
    c. tuna fish
    d. pork liver

38. Vitamin E helps in the metabolism of calcium and good sources are
    a. lean meats
    b. wheat germ
    c. legumes and nuts
    d. green leafy vegetables

39. Vitamin C is recommended for wound care patients as it
    a. helps the health of teeth and gums
    b. improves nerve functioning
    c. aids in wound healing
    d. is essential for maintaining strength of blood vessels

40. Alcoholics especially need thiamine (B_1) for its benefit of
    a. improved nerve functioning
    b. healthy appetite
    c. blood clotting
    d. carbohydrate metabolism

41. Vitamin B_1 is found in which foods?
    a. peanut butter
    b. enriched cereals
    c. liver and other organ meats
    d. wheat germ

42. Why should folic acid be included in a pregnant woman's diet?
    a. essential for formation of red blood cells
    b. shiny healthy hair and skin
    c. growth of bones and teeth
    d. protein metabolism

Meal Planning Exercise. *After reading the client stories, write a balanced meal plan for the requested meal.*

43. Mr. Eisenhower had a stroke three years ago and has mild dysphagia, difficulty swallowing. Breakfast is his favorite meal. What can he have for breakfast?

44. Mrs. Barber came from a farm family and is used to having dinner at lunchtime. She has congestive heart failure and is on a diuretic. What would you prepare for dinner?

45. Miss Sanchez loved to cook Spanish foods for dinner, but due to her chronic obstructive pulmonary disease she needs to wear oxygen and easily tires after a few bites. Dr. Arnold is concerned because she has lost 15 pounds in the past three months. Prepare a balanced meal plan for her.

46. Mr. Douglas has crippling rheumatoid arthritis, is wheelchair bound, and despite using eating utensils with built-up handles, he gets more food on the floor than in his mouth. He now needs assistance with eating. What would you prepare for lunch?

47. Mrs. Li is carrying triplets and is on bed rest for the next three weeks. What nutritious breakfast items should she have?

UNIT 13   ELIMINATION

LEARNING OBJECTIVES

After studying this unit, you should be able to:
- Describe organs and functions of the urinary tract system
- Discuss four urinary tract disorders
- Define the terms used to describe signs and symptoms of urinary disorders
- Describe three types of urinary incontinence
- Identify fluids that are recorded for intake and output
- List the reasons for recording fluid intake and output
- Demonstrate the following:
  Procedure 20   Measuring and Recording Fluid Intake and Output
  Procedure 21   Giving and Emptying the Bedpan
  Procedure 22   Giving and Emptying the Urinal
  Procedure 23   Assisting Client to Use the Portable Commode
  Procedure 24   Collecting a Clean-Catch Urine Specimen
  Procedure 25   Caring for a Urinary Catheter
  Procedure 26   Connecting the Leg Bag
  Procedure 27   Emptying a Drainage Unit
  Procedure 28   Applying a Condom (External) Catheter
  Procedure 29   Retraining the Bladder
  Procedure 30   Giving a Commercial Enema
  Procedure 31   Giving a Rectal Suppository
  Procedure 32   Regulating the Bowels
  Procedure 33   Applying Adult Briefs
  Procedure 34   Collecting a Stool Specimen
  Procedure 35   Assisting with Changing an Ostomy Bag

TERMS TO DEFINE

- bladder
- clean-catch specimen
- colonoscopy
- colostomy
- cystitis
- detrusor instability
- dysuria

- edema
- enema
- fluid balance
- frequency
- hematuria
- hemodialysis
- hesitancy

- impaction
- incontinent
- Kegel exercises
- kidneys
- kidney dialysis
- kidney stones
- meatus
- oliguria
- ostomy
- ostomy bag
- perineum

- peritoneal dialysis
- pyuria
- renal
- restricted fluids
- stoma
- suppository
- ureters
- urethra
- urgency
- urinary catheter

APPLICATION EXERCISES

Short Answer/Fill in the Blanks. *Complete the following sentences with the correct word or words.*

1. The urinary system is composed of the kidneys, ureters, _____, and urethra.

2. The primary organs of the urinary system are the _____, which filter waste material from the bloodstream.

3. The muscular organ for storing urine is called the _____.

4. The normal urine color is clear, _____ _____ with a mild _____ odor.

5. When the normal bladder contains about _____ to _____ cc of urine, a person has an urge to urinate or _____.

6. Signs and symptoms of urinary problems may include: _____, painful urination; _____, finding traces of blood in the urine; _____, voiding in small amounts; _____, going to the bathroom more often than usual and only voiding a small amount of urine; _____, inability to void; and _____, unable to control the flow of urine.

7. List three ways of preventing urinary tract infections.

    a. _____

    b. _____

    c. _____

8. Individuals who have lost control of the bladder are referred to as _____.

9. Involuntary loss of small amounts of urine during activities that increase intra-abdominal pressure such as coughing, running, laughing, or lifting heavy objects is called _____. Pelvic floor exercises known as _____ may improve this condition by tightening the muscles around the urinary meatus.

10. _____ _____ is usually caused by weakened pelvic floor muscles, tumor, bladder stones, or diverticuli.

11. Unstable bladder known as _____ _____ is associated with disorders of the lower urinary tract or neurological disorders including multiple sclerosis and diabetes.

12. Inflammation of the lining of the bladder is called _____. Signs and symptoms are urinary _____ and _____, dysuria, nausea, _____ (loss of appetite), and fever.

13. Incontinence of urine can cause skin _____.

14. Kidney stones can cause _____ urination. Signs and symptoms of renal colic are sudden severe pain in the _____ area, _____ due to stones trying to pass through the _____, nausea, and fever.

15. _____ _____ occurs when a client's kidneys no longer produce urine and waste products build up in the body; if nothing is done, the client can die.

16. Two treatments for renal failure are kidney _____ or kidney _____.

17. List the two types of kidney dialysis.

    a. _____

    b. _____

18. A measure of all the fluids or semiliquids that a person drinks is called _____.

19. The abbreviation for measuring fluid intake and fluid output is _____.

20. A _____ _____ _____ is requested to obtain a urine sample that is as free of contamination as possible.

21. A _____ _____ is a tube inserted into the bladder to drain urine.

22. The closed drainage system should _____ be disconnected except to connect to a leg bag.

23. A urinary leg bag allows the client greater _____ but must be emptied more often.

24. When the leg bag is not being used, it must be sealed with a clean _____ or _____.

25. The home health aide needs to keep a record of how often and how much a client _____ to learn the client's voiding patterns.

26. Bladder training includes offering the client a specified amount of fluid, and _____ minutes later, the aide should _____ the client.

27. During bladder training, the client needs _____ to remain dry.

28. A common cause of incontinence is _____ in getting to the bathroom.

29. The intervals between toileting may be _____ as control of the bladder is established.

30. An _____ is the technique of introducing fluid into the rectum to remove feces and flatus from the rectum and colon.

31. A _____ contains ingredients that once absorbed by the lining of the colon will stimulate the colon to evacuate stool.

32. Illness, poor eating habits, drug therapy, and lack of exercise can cause _____.

33. _____ is the unusual retention of fecal matter along with infrequent or difficult passage of stony, hard stool.

34. Important elements of a bowel regulating plan include:

    a. _____

    b. _____

    c. _____

    d. _____

    e. _____

    f. _____

    g. _____

35. A large amount of stool in the lower rectum or colon is called an _____.

36. An impaction must be removed by a _____.

37. To minimize embarrassment to the client in the event of an accident, the client can wear an _____ _____.

38. An operation in which the intestine is cut and brought to the outside of the body is called a _____ or an _____.

39. A client with a new colostomy needs the home health aide to be _____ and not show _____.

40. For the home health aide to irrigate a client's _____, the aide needs to have advanced training from the agency.

Multiple Choice. *Choose the correct answer or answers.*

41. Actions the home health aide can take to help the client who is constipated include

    a. encouraging fluid intake   c. encouraging exercise

    b. increasing fiber in diet   d. encouraging the use of laxatives

42. The purpose of caring properly for an ostomy bag is to

    a. keep the client clean   c. regulate daily routine for removing wastes

    b. prevent skin breakdown   d. all of these

43. The home health aide monitoring intake for a client needs to measure

    a. coffee   c. sugar

    b. cream   d. toast

44. Measures the home health aide can perform to prevent skin breakdown in the incontinent client include

    a. keeping the perineal area clean and dry   c. inspecting the affected area frequently

    b. applying moisture barrier ointment   d. changing the adult brief at least daily

45. When the membrane lining the bladder becomes inflamed, _____ occurs.

    a. incontinence   c. kidney stones

    b. cystitis   d. none of these

Documentation Exercises. *Read the following descriptions and provide documentation for each scenario.*

46. You have given your client a Fleet enema. His bowel movement was dark brown and very hard. He passed some flatus and stated he felt much better. Document this occurrence.

47. Your client is incontinent of urine frequently. She uses five to six adult briefs a day. How would you document this?

48. You have been asked to collect a urine specimen from your client. You have collected it. Document it.

Label the Diagram

49. Label the parts of the urinary system on the diagram; refer to Figure 13–1.

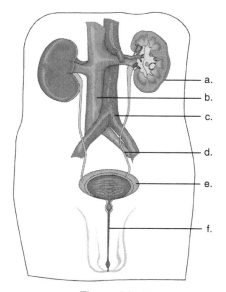

a. _____
b. _____
c. _____
d. _____
e. _____
f. _____

Figure 13–1

50. Record the oral intake of Mr. Zigouski on the form provided in Figure 13–2.
    The following cups, bowls, and glasses are used in the home:

juice glass	150 mL	carton of milk	240 mL
bowl	250 mL	custard, ice cream, and gelatin	125 mL
coffee cup	200 mL		

Mr. Zigouski's Meal Plan:

Breakfast:

1 glass apple juice   wheat bran cereal
1 carton milk   1/2 cup mixed berries

Lunch:

1 cup of coffee   1/2 cup applesauce
1 bowl of chicken and rice soup   turkey sandwich on white toast
lettuce and tomato salad

Dinner:

1 cup coffee   1 cup steamed vegetables
1 baked potato   1/c cup vanilla ice cream (container)
4 oz meatloaf

Intake Section of Intake and Output Form					
INTAKE					
Time	Oral		Tube Feeding	Intravenous	Other
	Kind	Amount			
8-Hour Total					
8-Hour Total					
8-Hour Total					
24-Hour Total					

Figure 13–2

51. Indicate with a yes or no which areas could be contaminated; refer to Figure 13–3.

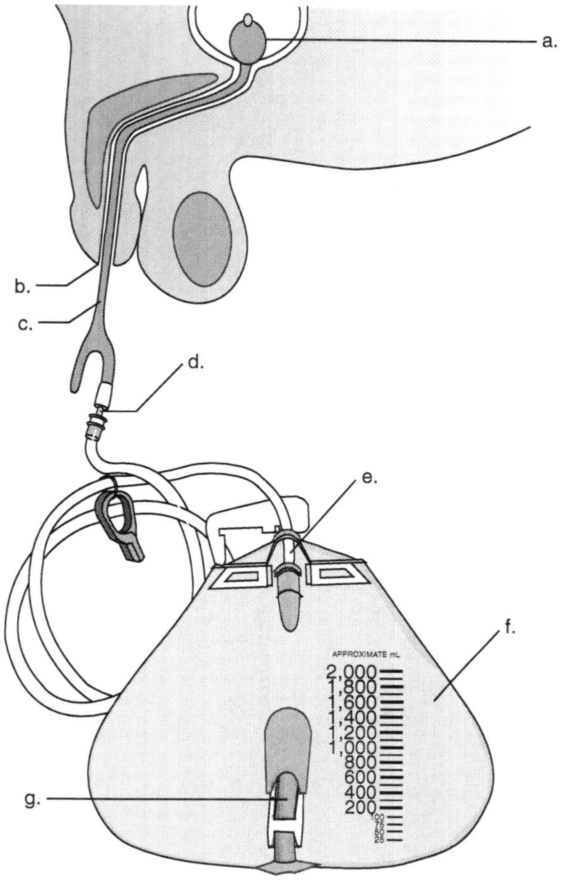

a. _____

b. _____

c. _____

d. _____

e. _____

f. _____

g. _____

Figure 13–3

52. Use the following measurements to fill out the urinary output portion of the I&O form in Figure 13–4.

0630 client voided 450 mL urine
0900 client voided 200 mL urine
1330 client voided 345 mL urine
1615 client voided 280 mL urine
2220 client voided 370 mL urine

Output Section of Intake and Output Form				
OUTPUT				
Time	Urine	Emesis	BM	Other/ Kind
8-Hour Total				
8-Hour Total				
8-Hour Total				
24-Hour Total				

Figure 13–4

PRACTICE SITUATIONS

Case 1

You have been assigned to care for Mrs. Schultz. She has an indwelling catheter. You are to give her a bath, prepare a meal, and change the bed linens. After you have bathed her and prepared her meal, you assist her into a wheelchair to eat. When you return to clean up her dishes, you notice urine on the floor. You know she has a catheter in place.

Questions

1. What would you check first?

2. What do you think is causing the leaking?

3. Do you need to notify anyone? If yes, who?

Case 2

You are working with Mr. Pipo and part of your assignment includes toilet training his bladder. You are to take him to the toilet every two hours. You have been doing this for more than a week. He seems to understand, but when you take him to the toilet, he cannot urinate. When you return him to bed, he urinates on the floor.

Questions

1. What do you think is going on?

2. Do you think he is purposely not cooperating?

3. Can you talk to him about the problem?

CROSSWORD PUZZLE

Across

5 involuntary loss of urine during activities

6 opening into the urethra

7 inflammation of the diverticula in colon

9 exercises that strengthen pelvic muscles

12 difficulty urinating

13 artificial opening into body to drain wastes

14 muscular organ for storing urine

15 frequent urination

Down

1 tube inserted into the bladder to drain urine

2 bloody urine

3 intake of fluids limited

4 hard stool in the lower rectum

8 tube passages draining urine from kidney to bladder

10 cone-shaped, medicated mass that facilitates a bowel movement on insertion

11 appliance to contain waste products

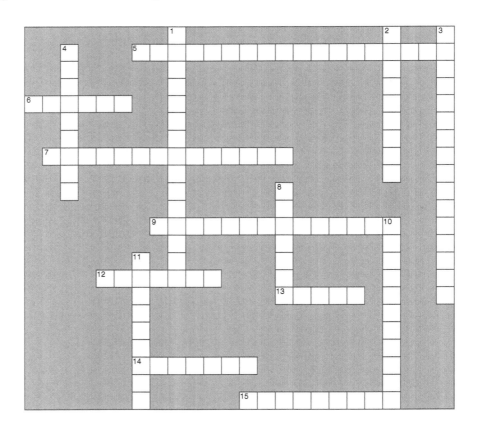

UNIT QUIZ

Short Answer/Fill in the Blanks. *Complete the following sentences with the correct word or words.*

1. The kidneys, ureters, bladder, and urethra make up the _____ _____.

2. The _____ filter waste material from the bloodstream.

3. List five signs and symptoms of urinary problems.

   a. _____

   b. _____

   c. _____

   d. _____

   e. _____

4. The daily output of urine is _____ to _____ cc.

5. Painful urination and flank pain are signs of _____ _____.

6. _____ is a decrease in the amount of water in the body tissues due to insufficient intake of fluids or excretion of excess fluids.

7. Swelling of body tissues with water retained by the body is called _____.

8. Fluid balance means that the client _____ about the same amount of fluid that is taken _____.

9. _____ is the measurement of fluid taken in by the body while _____ is fluid eliminated from the body and recorded.

10. Five fluids that should be included in the measurement of intake and output include:

    a. _____

    b. _____

    c. _____

    d. _____

    e. _____

11. List four items that need to be measured for output.

    a. _____

    b. _____

    c. _____

    d. _____

12. Clients with _____ _____ have no voluntary control of their bladder muscles and expel urine unexpectedly.

13. List three characteristics of normal urine.

    a. _____

    b. _____

    c. _____

14. Care of the client with an indwelling catheter is aimed at preventing _____.

15. _____ _____ refers to involuntary urination because of inability to reach a bathroom due to physical disability, inaccessible toilet, or inattentive caregivers.

16. A _____ is used for clients who are confined to bed and should be _____ whenever the client requests it.

17. Stool or feces should be observed for:

    a. _____

    b. _____

    c. _____

18. Constipation often occurs among older adults due to lack of _____, or moving about regularly, and pain _____.

19. An _____ is a large amount of hard stool in the lower colon or _____ that cannot be expelled normally.

20. The purpose of a commercial enema is to cleanse the _____.

21. Oil-retention enemas are given to _____ _____ _____.

22. An adult brief is used to keep the incontinent client _____ and to minimize _____ to the client in the event of _____.

23. A _____ is an artificial opening into the large intestine with the stool usually formed; an _____ is an artificial opening into the small intestine with a more liquid and odorous stool.

24. After colostomy surgery, the opening in the abdomen is called a _____ with the _____ _____ placed over the opening to collect wastes.

25. An ostomy bag should be emptied when it becomes _____ to _____ full.

Matching. *Match each definition with the correct term.*

26. _____ painful urination

27. _____ finding traces of blood in the urine

28. _____ voiding in small amounts

29. _____ going to the bathroom frequently and only voiding a small amount of urine

30. _____ inability to void

31. _____ no voluntary control of bladder muscles, expel urine unexpectedly

32. _____ pain in the area between the ribs and hip bone in the client's back

33. _____ delay in starting to void

34. _____ urine comes out slower or at different rates

35. _____ having pus in the urine

36. _____ having to void immediately

37. _____ unable to control the flow of urine when sneezing or coughing

38. _____ perineal area

39. _____ portable toilet

40. _____ in-toilet specimen container

a. change in stream of urine

b. commode

c. dysuria

d. flank pain

e. frequency

f. hematuria

g. hesitancy

h. incontinent

i. oliguria

j. perineum

k. potty hat

l. pyuria

m. retention

n. stress incontinence

o. urgency

Multiple Choice. *Choose the correct answer or answers.*

41. What is the purpose of keeping the catheter collection bag below the level of the urinary bladder?

    a. assist the gravity drainage

    b. prevent backflow of urine into the bladder

    c. prevent bag from being slept on

    d. easily visible to members of health care team for assessment

42. Catheter care should be performed by

    a. using soap and warm water or antiseptic wipes

    b. using antibiotic wipes

    c. wiping the catheter tube starting at the urinary opening and wiping away from it

    d. wiping the catheter tube starting at connection site to catheter bag and wipe toward urinary opening

43. When performing catheter care, which observations need to be reported to the nurse?

    a. bleeding

    b. crusting

    c.   use of skin barrier ointment

    d.   dark yellow, foul urine

44. A condom catheter is used to

    a. help cleanse the bowels

    b. prevent skin breakdown in incontinent male

    c. prevent skin breakdown in incontinent female

    d. drain urine from the urethra through a tube to a drainage receptacle

45. The medical term for having a bowel movement is

    a. flatus

    b. diverticulitis

    c.   constipation

    d.   defecation

46. Three common disorders of the lower intestines and rectum are

    a. kidney stones

    b. diverticulitis

    c.   hemorrhoids

    d.   cancer of the colon

47. Mr. Putnam had a stroke and constipation developed. A bowel regulating program was developed. This involves

    a. setting up a designated time for a bowel movement

    b. eating foods that are high in fiber and bulk

    c. drinking eight glasses of water a day

    d. all of the above

48. Miss Marchetti has urinary frequency and urgency, dysuria, nausea, and anorexia. Her temperature is 101.6°F. She has signs of

    a. kidney stones

    b. stress incontinence

    c.   renal failure

    d.   cystitis

49. Mrs. Hamilton has had hypertension for 20 years. She has been weak and tired with increased lethargy over the past six months. Increasing ankle edema, abdominal bloating, and fluid retention have occurred. Her health care provider states she needs dialysis. Mrs. Hamilton has developed

    a. kidney stones

    b. stress incontinence

    c.   renal failure

    d.   cystitis

50. Mr. Lightfoot has had diarrhea, abdominal cramping, and increased rectal gas for the past three months. He saw a gastroenterologist who performed a colonoscopy. The biopsy for cancer was negative. The gastroenterologist diagnosed

    a. diverticulitis

    b. hemorrhoids

    c.   colon cancer

    d.   flatulence

UNIT 14   INTEGUMENTARY SYSTEM

LEARNING OBJECTIVES

After studying this unit, you should be able to:
- Identify parts and functions of the integumentary system
- Describe common skin disorders
- Describe the appearance of pressure sores
- Locate the pressure point on the body where pressure sores usually occur
- Describe nursing measures to prevent pressure sores from developing
- List guidelines for application of ointment to the skin
- Demonstrate the following:
  Procedure 36   Applying Clean Dressing and Ointment to Broken Skin
  Procedure 37   Assisting with Tub Bath or Shower
  Procedure 38   Giving a Bed Bath
  Procedure 39   Giving a Back Rub
  Procedure 40   Giving Female Perineal Care
  Procedure 41   Giving Male Perineal Care
  Procedure 42   Assisting with Routine Oral Hygiene
  Procedure 43   Caring for Dentures
  Procedure 44   Shaving the Male Client
  Procedure 45   Performing a Warm Foot Soak
  Procedure 46   Giving Nail Care
  Procedure 47   Shampooing Hair in Bed

TERMS TO DEFINE

- bony prominence
- dermis
- epidermis
- podiatrist
- pressure sores

APPLICATION EXERCISES

Short Answer/Fill in the Blanks. *Complete the following sentences with the correct word or words.*

1. The integumentary system is made up of the skin, _____, and
   _____.

2. Skin is the _____ organ of the body, made up of two layers: the outer layer is
   the _____ and the inner layer is the _____.

143

3. Three functions of the skin are:

   a. _____

   b. _____

   c. _____

4. The natural openings in the skin are called _____.

5. Secretions from the glands help keep _____ from entering the pores.

6. The pus that forms on a skin wound is made up of _____
   _____ _____ _____ that have fought off
   germs.

7. Three ways that hair protects the body are:

   a. _____

   b. _____

   c. _____

8. A person who gets little exercise and spends most of the time lying in the same place can
   expect to experience _____ _____.

9. Skin breakdown is most likely to occur over _____ _____.

10. Six areas of the body that are likely to experience skin breakdown are:

    a. _____

    b. _____

    c. _____

    d. _____

    e. _____

    f. _____

11. Describe the four stages of pressure sores.

    a. _____

    b. _____

    c. _____

    d. _____

12. The home health aide needs to reposition the bedridden client _____ to
    prevent skin breakdown.

13. Four components of good skin care that the home health aide must perform are:

    a. _____

    b. _____

    c. _____

    d. _____

14. Many special devices are available to place on the bed or on the specific part of the body to
    aid in prevention of _____ _____. Examples of these are air
    pressure mattress, gel foam cushion for wheelchairs, _____ mattress or
    cushion, lamb's wool or _____ pads, bed cradle, elbow pads,
    _____ pads, and ankle elevators.

15. Home health aides are allowed to apply over-the-counter ointments to _____ skin areas.

16. List three things home health aides must do when applying over-the-counter ointments.

    a. _____

    b. _____

    c. _____

17. Good hygiene is important to maintain _____ integrity, prevent _____, and to refresh and _____ the client.

18. List four common skin disorders.

    a. _____

    b. _____

    c. _____

    d. _____

19. The home health aide should check the client's skin for any signs of _____ when giving a bath.

20. The purposes of giving the client a bed bath include cleaning the client, _____, _____, and observing the body for signs of _____ _____.

21. A back rub is given to increase the blood _____ to the back and to provide _____ and _____ to the client.

22. The area from the genitals to the anus is called the _____.

23. Good oral hygiene is important to keep the client's _____ and _____ healthy.

24. Personal care includes _____, nail care, and _____.

True or False. *Answer the following statements true (T) or false (F).*

25. T   F   The skin is the largest organ of the body.

26. T   F   Scabies is a chronic inflammatory disease of the oil glands and hair follicles.

27. T   F   The home health aide needs to inform the nurse when the client's skin breakdown has reached a Stage 3.

28. T   F   If the client is left lying in a urine-soaked bed, the skin breakdown will occur rapidly.

29. T   F   If the client is lying in a bed with an air mattress, it is not necessary to turn the client every two hours.

30. T   F   To prevent cuts, clients on blood thinners should not use a regular razor.

31. T   F   Bathwater should be around 120°F and tub should be 3/4 filled for bathing.

32. T   F   Use a soft toothbrush of toothette to clean a client's mouth while dentures are soaking.

33. T   F   Best practice is to use an electric heating pad set on high and placed on the client's abdomen.

34. T   F   It is a good idea to offer the client the bedpan before giving a bath.

35. T   F   Keeping the perineum clean is important to prevent infection.

Matching. *Match each term with the correct definition.*

36. _____ air mattress

37. _____ eggcrate

38. _____ sheepskin

39. _____ gel foam

40. _____ heel pads

41. _____ water mattress

a. barrier between the client's skin and the sheets

b. mattress filled with air

c. special cushion filled with a solution or gel

d. mattress filled with water

e. foam waffled mattress

f. special protectors for the heel

Multiple Choice. *Choose the correct answer or answers.*

42. Areas of the body especially prone to the skin breakdown include

a. bony prominences

b. areas covered with hair

c. urine-soaked areas

d. a and c only

43. Special devices that can help prevent skin breakdown include

a. cane

b. walker

c. wheelchair

d. sheepskin and elbow and heel pads

44. The home health aide performing dressing changes needs to document the

a. size of the wound

b. color of the drainage

c. color of the bandage used

d. a and b only

45. The purpose of giving the client a bed bath is to

a. provide exercise for the aide

b. put the client at ease

c. clean and refresh the client

d. give the client an opportunity to talk

46. The bedpan should be offered

a. before bathing

b. after eating

c. before ambulating the client

d. all of these

Documentation Exercises. *Read the following descriptions and provide documentation for each scenario.*

47. Your client has a wound on his lower left leg. You are required to perform a dressing change. You notice the wound is approximately 1 inch in diameter and is a very dark red. You apply antibiotic ointment, a sterile 4 × 4 gauze pad, and tape to secure. Document this.

48. Caring for your client includes giving a bed bath, making the bed, and transforming the client into a wheelchair. How would you document his care?

49. When you arrive to care for Mr. Moon, you find him sitting outside in the sun. The weather is very hot. He tells you that he feels terrible. He is dizzy, nauseated, and feels very weak. His skin is very dry, and he has chest pain. After you call for help, what do you document?

Label the Diagram

50. Refer to Figure 14–1 and draw a circle around 10 areas at-risk for the development of pressure ulcers.

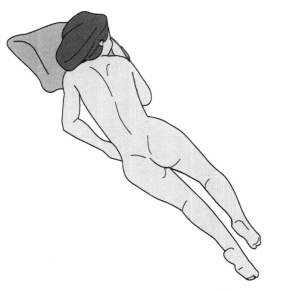

Figure 14–1

51. Indicate with a yes or no whether the diagram shows the correct taping; refer to Figure 14–2.

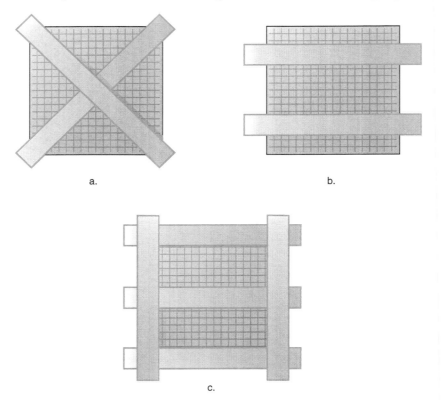

a.

b.

c.

Figure 14–2

a. _____

b. _____

c. _____

52. Label the parts of the integumentary system; refer to Figure 14–3.

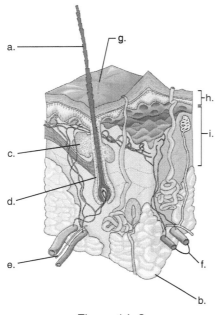

Figure 14–3

a. _____

b. _____

c. _____

d. _____

e. _____

f. _____

g. _____

h. _____

i. _____

PRACTICE SITUATIONS

Case 1

Mrs. Rizzo has been your client for several months. She has had a stroke and is unable to turn in bed without your assistance. You have tried consistently to keep her off her back, but she will wiggle and squirm in the bed until she is back on her back. Today when you are bathing her, you notice broken skin on her coccyx.

Questions

1. What do you do?

2. What can you tell her?

3. Who do you contact?

4. How do you care for the area with broken skin?

Case 2

You have given your client a bath and dressed her in clean clothes. You go to the kitchen to prepare food. When you return, you find she has removed all of her clothing.

Questions

1. What do you think caused her to do this?

2. What do you do?

3. How can you prevent this from happening again?

CROSSWORD PUZZLE

Across

4 skin covering the bones

5 skin lesions caused by mites

9 synthetic or wool pressure relieving device

10 inner layer of skin

12 air-inflated pressure relieving device

Down

1 waffled pressure relieving device

2 doctor specializing in foot and ankle care

3 skin inflammation causes itching, redness, and skin lesions

6 breakdown of skin over bony area

7 chronic inflammatory disease of the oil glands and hair follicles

8 scaly, itchy skin eruptions

11 pressure sore measurement

13 outer layer of skin

14 largest organ of the body

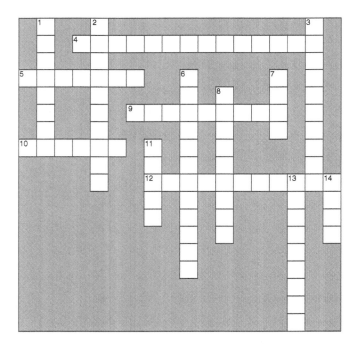

UNIT QUIZ

Short Answer/Fill in the Blanks. *Complete the following sentences with the correct word or words.*

1. The skin, hair, and nails make up the _____ system.

2. The largest organ of the body is the _____.

3. The skin is made up of two layers: _____ and _____.

4. The skin is a protective covering that helps

   a. _____

   b. _____

   c. _____

5. Certain medical conditions make the client more susceptible to skin breakdown such as _____, stroke, paralysis, client with _____ problems, and clients who are obese or very thin.

6. Oil glands and sweat glands produce secretions that are helpful in keeping _____ from entering the pores.

7. As the body perspires through the skin pores, the air evaporates the perspiration and the body feels _____.

8. When the body gets little exercise, the _____ is one of the first areas to break down, often occurring over the _____ _____.

9. List six areas of the body that are prone to skin breakdown.

   a. _____

   b. _____

   c. _____

   d. _____

   e. _____

   f. _____

10. Home health aides are an important part of a bedridden client's pressure sore prevention program by providing excellent skin _____, turning and repositioning the client _____, and performing range-of-motion exercises.

11. The incontinent client's skin care includes _____ at the time of soiling, applying moisture barrier _____, and the use of underpads or adult briefs that absorb moisture.

12. Pressure sores are characterized by _____, depending on the degree of severity.

13. List four pressure reduction devices.

   a. _____

   b. _____

   c. _____

   d. _____

14. Sheepskin or lamb's wool pads prevent pressure ulcers by acting as a _____ between the client's skin and the sheets and reducing friction.

15. When applying braces and splints, the home health aide should watch for _____ _____ and immediately report the first sign of _____ skin to the nurse.

True or False. *Answer the following statements true (T) or false (F).*

16. T   F   Pressure sores are due to infection in the skin.

17. T   F   Secretions from the oil and sweat glands help keep germs from entering the body.

18. T   F   The diabetic client's nails may be trimmed by the home health aide.

19. T   F   Home health aides are permitted to apply prescription ointments to nonintact skin.

20. T   F   Always wear gloves when applying ointments so as not to absorb them into your own body.

21. T   F   A Stage 1 pressure sore involves blister formation and small breaks in the skin.

21. T   F   In a Stage 4 pressure ulcer, the open area extends to the muscles, bone, and underlying structures.

22. T   F   Recording drainage amounts is not needed, just the wound appearance and wound care provided are documented in the home health aide's notes.

23. T   F   Always wash your hands and apply gloves before starting wound care.

24. T   F   Vigorously massage reddened skin with lotion or barrier ointment.

25. T   F   Always apply a thick layer of ointment to protect the skin.

Matching. *Match each term with the correct definition.*

26. _____ pores
27. _____ pus
28. _____ dermis
29. _____ epidermis
30. _____ hair
31. _____ oil and sweat glands

a. natural openings in the skin
b. dead white blood cells that fought off germs
c. outer layer of skin
d. inner layer of skin
e. prevents small particles from entering nose and ears
f. helps to regulate body temperature

Multiple Choice. *Choose the correct answer or answers.*

32. Pressure ulcers most often form over
    a. trunk and back
    b. ankles and heels
    c. knees and hips
    d. nose and cheek

33. Common causes of pressure sore development are
    a. periods of inactivity
    b. urinary and fecal incontinence
    c. friction and shearing when turning
    d. all of the above

34. A chronic inflammatory disease of the oil glands and hair follicles characterized by eruptions, cysts, nodules, or pustules that may lead to scarring and pitting of the skin is called

    a. acne

    b. psoriasis

    c. dermatitis

    d. scabies

35. Skin condition that develops skin lesions caused by mites that burrow into the skin is known as

    a. acne

    b. psoriasis

    c. dermatitis

    d. scabies

36. This skin inflammation causes itching, redness, and skin lesions and is often caused by poison ivy, allergies, and sunburn

    a. acne

    b. psoriasis

    c. dermatitis

    d. scabies

37. Scaly, itchy skin eruptions that appear at any age, often seen at elbows and knees

    a. acne

    b. psoriasis

    c. dermatitis

    d. scabies

38. Skin care performed by home health aides should include

    a. washing the skin with warm water and mild soap and rinsing well, or using bag baths

    b. applying good moisturizing lotion to dry skin surfaces

    c. changing the incontinent client's soiled garments promptly

    d. all of the above

39. Examples of pressure relieving devices include

    a. alternating air mattress

    b. casts

    c. lamb's wool or sheepskin pad

    d. splints

40. Good pressure relieving devices for a client who sits in a wheelchair include

    a. eggcrate chair cushion

    b. gel cushion

    c. low air loss mattress

    d. ankle elevator

41. Home health aides need to report the following to the nurse

    a. redness or open areas underneath splints

    b. prolonged redness of skin

    c. patients found repeatedly in excessive soiled adult briefs

    d. all of the above

UNIT 15 MUSCULOSKELETAL SYSTEM: ARTHRITIS, BODY MECHANICS, AND RESTORATIVE CARE

LEARNING OBJECTIVES

After studying this unit, you should be able to:

- Identify components of the musculoskeletal system
- List three functions of the musculoskeletal system
- List four disorders of the musculoskeletal system and their main signs and symptoms
- Differentiate between the following three types of arthritis: rheumatoid, osteoarthritis, and gout
- Describe the nursing care given to clients with arthritis
- Explain nursing care for a client with a recent hip or knee replacement
- Explain the purposes for proper body mechanics
- List 10 rules of good body mechanics
- Identify comfort and safety measures for lifting, turning, and moving clients
- Explain the use of the gait or transfer belt
- Describe the term *dangling* a client
- Describe components of various mechanical lifts
- Identify comfort, alignment, and safety measures for positioning clients in bed
- Describe four different body positions that clients can be placed in
- Describe nursing care for a client with a leg cast
- Explain the purpose of applying cold to a body part
- Describe how to dress and undress a client with right-sided weakness
- Explain two complications of immobility
- Distinguish between active and passive range-of-motion exercises
- Demonstrate the following:
  Procedure 48   Applying a Transfer or Gait Belt
  Procedure 49   Dangling a Client
  Procedure 50   Turning the Client Toward You
  Procedure 51   Moving the Client Up in Bed Using the Drawsheet
  Procedure 52   Log Rolling the Client
  Procedure 53   Positioning the Client in Supine Position
  Procedure 54   Positioning the Client in Lateral/Side-Lying Position
  Procedure 55   Positioning the Client in Prone Position
  Procedure 56   Positioning the Client in Fowler's Position

TERMS TO DEFINE

- abduction
- active range-of-motion exercises
- activities
- adduction
- ambulate
- anti-inflammatory
- arthritis
- arthroplasty
- atrophy
- base of support
- body mechanics
- bursitis
- closed fracture
- contracture
- cyanosis
- dangle
- degenerative disease
- dorsiflexion
- extension
- external rotation
- flexion
- Fowler's position
- fracture
- gait belt
- gout
- internal rotation

- ligaments
- open fracture
- opposition
- osteoarthritis
- passive range-of-motion exercises
- pivot
- plantar flexion
- pronation
- prone position
- prostheses
- range-of-motion exercises
- rehabilitation
- rheumatoid arthritis
- rotation
- Sims' position
- sprain
- stand lift
- steroids
- supination
- synchronize
- tendon
- tophi
- total hip replacement
- total knee replacement
- transfer belt

APPLICATION EXERCISES

Short Answer/Fill in the Blanks. *Complete the following sentences with the correct word or words.*

1. The musculoskeletal system is made up of _____ and _____, which protect the internal _____ _____ and make _____ _____ possible.

2. The protective covering of the brain is called the _____.

3. Tough elastic fibers that hold the bones together are called _____.

4. The _____ allow the bones to be moved in certain ways.

5. The elbows and knees have hinge joints, which move in only _____ directions.

6. Joints at the shoulder and pelvis are _____ and _____ joints, which allow circular movement.

7. The wrist, ankles, and spinal column have _____ joints that allow only a limited sliding motion.

8. Muscles whose movement is controlled by the brain are called _____ muscles.

9. The heart is an example of an _____ muscle because it works automatically without any conscious effort by the individual.

10. The most common musculoskeletal problems are injuries caused by _____.

11. A break in a bone is called a _____. A _____ fracture is a break in the bone but not in the skin, while an _____ fracture occurs when the bone is fractured and the skin is broken.

12. Partial tearing of a muscle, tendon, or ligament due to trauma is a _____.

13. Affecting _____ of persons over age 65, _____ involves joint inflammation producing painful, swollen, and enlarged joints.

14. The two most common types of arthritis are:

    a. _____

    b. _____

15. The most difficult time of day for clients with rheumatoid arthritis is the _____.

16. List four major warning signs of inflammatory arthritis.

    a. _____

    b. _____

    c. _____

    d. _____

17. "Wear and tear" arthritis affects the weight-bearing joints such as spine, hip, and knees and is known as _____.

18. A type of arthritis that affects mainly men over age 40 is called _____ and is due to the presence of too much uric acid.

19. The first sign of gout is a painful _____ _____; other joints that may be affected such as the foot, ankle, and wrist may have little outpouches or protruding lesions called _____ that contain abnormal amounts of uric acid.

20. Arthritis is managed with _____ therapy, an _____ program, surgery, and _____.

21. Clients with arthritis may have lack of appetite because of _____.

22. If the client is experiencing pain in the joints, it is a good idea to remind the client to take pain medicine a half-hour before performing _____.

23. Decreased activity may cause the arthritic client to _____ weight.

24. Impaired _____ may cause lack of energy for preparing foods and shopping by the client with arthritis.

25. Aspirin is the drug of choice for arthritis, but sometimes it causes problems with the person's _____.

26. The largest group of drugs now used to treat arthritis are called _____ _____ drugs (NSAIDs), which work by decreasing pain and swelling in the joints and muscles.

27. The client who uses many over-the-counter medications to treat arthritic pain should be encouraged to contact his or her _____ regarding medications.

28. Side effects of arthritis drugs are: _____ _____, bloody urine, ringing in the ears, and _____ _____, which the home health aide needs to report to the nurse if observed or reported by the client.

29. The most powerful drugs used to treat arthritis are called _____, which can cause edema, _____ _____, susceptibility to infections and elevated blood pressure.

30. Four symptoms of rheumatoid arthritis are:

    a. _____

    b. _____

    c. _____

    d. _____

31. Assistive devices are used to maintain _____, simplify _____, and minimize _____ to the joints.

32. Correct positioning of the body can make the client _____ and assist the body to _____ more efficiently.

33. Four symptoms of osteoarthritis are:

    a. _____

    b. _____

    c. _____

    d. _____

34. Many times the client with arthritis can be helped by _____.

35. Surgical replacement of a joint is called _____.

36. Joint replacement surgery involves replacing a damaged or worn-out joint with an artificial part called a _____.

37. Five guidelines for caring for a client with new hip or knee replacement are:

    a. _____

    b. _____

    c. _____

    d. _____

    e. _____

38. After surgery, a device used to help the client breathe more deeply is called an

    _____ _____.

39. Casts are used to immobilize _____ or joints after trauma.

40. In caring for clients with casts, you examine the cast for signs of _____ that may cause skin irritation.

41. List four important aspects of caring for casts.

    a. _____

    b. _____

    c. _____

    d. _____

42. The way in which the body moves and keeps its balance through the use of all its parts is referred to as _____ _____.

43. It is important for home health aides to use _____ _____, which makes lifting, pulling, and pushing easier.

44. Avoid twisting your body as you work and bend, _____ the whole body instead.

45. List five basic rules of good body mechanics to prevent injury and reduce fatigue.

    a. _____

    b. _____

    c. _____

    d. _____

    e. _____

46. The home health aide should apply the following five techniques of good body mechanics while working:

    a. _____

    b. _____

    c. _____

    d. _____

    e. _____

47. If an unsteady client starts to fall, you should _____ _____ client to the _____.

48. The purpose of using a transfer or gait belt is to:

    a. _____

    b. _____

49. Dangling the client after surgery is done to move the client's legs around to prevent
_____ _____ and to _____
_____ on the client's back.

50. When dangling the patient, check the client's _____ to see if it is strong. If
client becomes faint, tip the _____ _____
_____ for a few seconds.

51. When the client is turned on the side, check to see if the _____ and
_____ are in correct alignment.

52. When moving the client up in bed, use a _____ to move the client with
minimum discomfort.

53. After spinal injury or hip fractures, _____ _____ a client to
ensure the spinal column is kept straight.

54. Proper _____ can relieve pressure on body parts, aid in breathing, as well as
preventing _____ to the client.

55. Range-of-motion exercises are performed on clients to _____
_____ from happening.

56. If the client can do range-of-motion exercises without the assistance of another person, they
are called _____ range-of-motion exercises; if performed with support of
another person, they are called _____ range-of-motion exercises.

57. Guidelines for doing range-of-motion exercises include:

    a. _____

    b. _____

    c. _____

    d. _____

    e. _____

58. _____ is the restoring of physical abilities to the highest level possible.

59. Before a home health aide assists in a rehabilitation program, he or she must be instructed by
a nurse or _____ _____.

60. A cane is used primarily for _____, while a _____ is used to
provide maximum stability as a client moves.

61. The home health aide should report to the case manager, nurse, or physical therapist any
client's lack of _____ or interest in a therapy program.

True or False. *Answer the following statements true (T) or false (F).*

62. T F There are more than 200 bones in the body.

63. T F Involuntary muscles are controlled by the brain.

64. T F The interior of the bone produces new blood cells for the circulatory system.

65. T F The heart is an example of a voluntary muscle.

66. T F Involuntary muscles form the walls of organs and these muscles work automatically.

67. T F Arthritis is seen more often in the elderly.

68. T F Arthritis affects 50% of the people over the age of 65, and men are affected twice as
often as women.

69. T   F   Rheumatoid arthritis affects all ages.

70. T   F   Arthritis is a chronic degenerative disease.

71. T   F   Exercises that the client can perform without assistance are referred to as passive range-of-motion exercises.

72. T   F   The goal of an exercise program includes maintaining joint movement or increasing joint movement.

73. T   F   If the client with arthritis has an exercise program, it is important for the program to be followed by the client even if it is painful.

74. T   F   It is important for the aide to be able to position the client's body correctly.

75. T   F   If the client with a cast develops a crack in the cast, the aide should tape it with adhesive tape.

76. T   F   Heat applications can increase circulation to a body part.

Matching. *Match each term with the correct definition.*

77. _____	abduction	a. touch each fingertip with the thumb
78. _____	adduction	b. to move a body part away from the midline of the body
79. _____	dorsiflexion	
80. _____	extension	c. straighten out a joint
81. _____	flexion	d. turning palms upward
82. _____	opposition	e. turning a joint inward
83. _____	internal rotation	f. to move a body part toward the midline of the body
84. _____	external rotation	
85. _____	planter flexion	g. turning a joint in a circle
86. _____	pronation	h. bending foot toward ankle
87. _____	rotation	i. bend a joint
88. _____	supination	j. turning a joint outward
		k. bending the foot downward
		l. turning palms downward

Multiple Choice. *Choose the correct answer or answers.*

89. Surgery for arthritis can be performed on the following joints
    a. knee, hip, jaw
    b. spine, shoulder, finger
    c. hip, spine, wrist
    d. all of these

90. You assist the client to a sitting position. You need to check to see that
    a. the client has good body alignment
    b. the client can see the TV
    c. the clothes are clean and neat
    d. the client is relaxed

91. When you are making an occupied bed, you
    a. take all the sheets off before putting clean sheets on the bed
    b. ask the client to get out of the bed
    c. work on only one side of the bed at a time
    d. hurry through changing the bed so that you can get on with other tasks

92. Positioning clients in the Fowler's position
    a. helps assist them to breathe easier
    b. makes it easier for them to get out of bed
    c. allows you to change the bed easier
    d. none of these

93. During the procedure of transferring the client to a wheelchair, you
    a. press your knee against the client's stronger knee
    b. set the chair at a 90° angle to the bed
    c. press your knee against the client's weakest knee
    d. keep your feet together and flex your knees and hips

94. The purpose of applying a cold application to the client's skin is to
    a. ease pain
    b. numb the skin to dermis layer
    c. decrease swelling of localized area
    d. increase circulation to the area

95. When applying an ice application
    a. warm ice pack in the microwave
    b. always cover ice pack with a cloth
    c. always apply ice directly to the skin
    d. leave ice pack on for 20 minutes but check the client's skin every 5 minutes for redness, whiteness, or blue color

96. A patient who is partial weight-bearing, applies weight
    a. partially on the arms and unaffected leg
    b. all weight is placed on arms and unaffected leg
    c. minimally to the toes
    d. mostly on the arms and unaffected leg

97. Which assistive device is initially used to ambulate by a client who had a hip replacement?
    a. four-point cane
    b. crutches
    c. cane
    d. walker

98. When assisting a client who has poor balance to walk with a cane, the aide should
    a. support the strong side
    b. encourage the client to walk alone with the cane
    c. support the weak side
    d. encourage the client to use a walker instead

99. The home health aide performing range-of-motion exercises for the knee and hip should
    a. stand on the side being exercised
    b. support the calf and the toes
    c. support underneath the knee and ankle
    d. bend the knee and raise it to the chest

100. The exercise in which you face the wall, place one hand on the wall, bring back opposite leg as far as you can, hold for 10 seconds, and repeat with other leg is called
    a. hip adductor
    b. calf stretch
    c. hamstring stretch
    d. lower back stretch

Documentation Exercises. *Read the following descriptions and provide documentation for each scenario.*

101. You are assigned to Mrs. Howe, who has rheumatoid arthritis. You are instructed to give her a partial bed bath, allowing her to do as much as she is able to. When you give her the bath, she is only able to bathe her face and hands. Document her care.

102. You are assigned to ambulate Mrs. Geever, perform range-of-motion exercises to the lower extremities, and assist her to the bedside commode. Mrs. Geever complains of severe pain in her shoulder when you are assisting her to the bedside commode. She urinates a small amount and you return her to bed. Document your care and observations.

Label the Diagram

103. Label the parts of the muscular system on the diagram; refer to Figure 15–1.

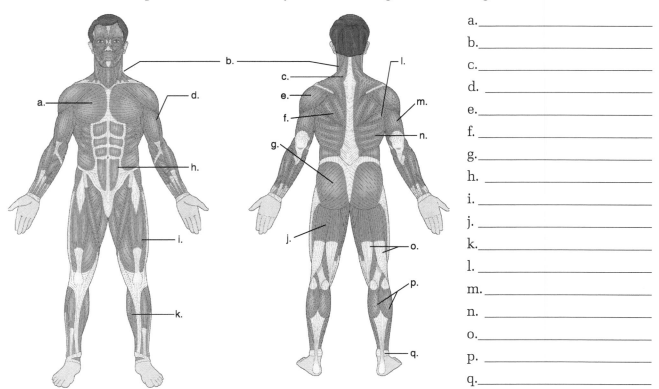

a._____

b._____

c._____

d. _____

e._____

f. _____

g._____

h. _____

i. _____

j. _____

k._____

l. _____

m._____

n. _____

o._____

p. _____

q._____

Figure 15–1

104. Review Figure 15–2. Choose the word for the range-of-motion exercises being performed:
    a. rotated
    b. adducted
    c. flexed
    d. abducted

105. Review Figure 15–3. Choose the word for the range-of-motion exercises being performed:
    a. rotated
    b. adducted
    c. flexed
    d. abducted

106. Review Figure 15–4. Choose the word for the range-of-motion exercises being performed:
    a. rotated
    b. adducted
    c. flexed
    d. abducted

107. Review Figure 15–5. Choose the word for the range-of-motion exercises being performed:
    a. rotated
    b. adducted
    c. flexed
    d. abducted

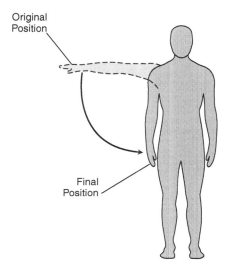

Figure 15–2

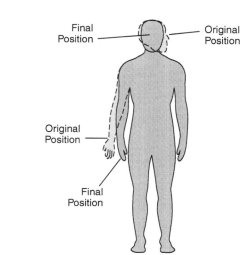

Figure 15–3

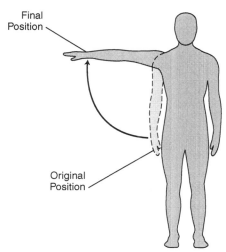

Figure 15–4

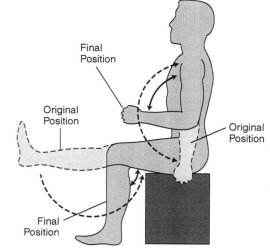

Figure 15–5

108. Label the parts of the skeletal system on the diagram; refer to Figure 15–6.

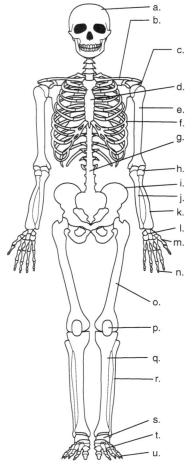

a. _____

b. _____

c. _____

d. _____

e. _____

f. _____

g. _____

h. _____

i. _____

j. _____

k. _____

l. _____

m. _____

n. _____

o. _____

p. _____

q. _____

r. _____

s. _____

t. _____

u. _____

Figure 15–6

PRACTICE SITUATIONS

Case 1

Your client, Mrs. Rodriguez, has severe arthritis. Part of your assignment is to perform range-of-motion exercises to her extremities. You also need to bathe her and straighten up her room.

Questions

1. What time do you think would be the best time to perform these exercises?

2. Is there anything you can do to make these exercises less painful to Mrs.Rodriguez?

Case 2

You have been assigned a new client, Mrs. Peltier. Your care plan includes giving her a bath and to help her into a wheelchair. When you arrive, you find Mrs. Peltier is bedridden and unable to assist with her care. She weighs in excess of 300 pounds. You will not be able to move her alone.

Questions

1. What can you do?
2. Is there anyone who can help you?
3. How could this have been avoided?

CROSSWORD PUZZLE

Across

2 medication to relieve pain and inflammation

4 break in the bone but not in the skin

6 type of arthritis due to increased uric acid

7 position on back with head of bed at 45° angle

10 walking with client

12 hanging legs loose over the outside of the bed

13 turning to the side instead of twisting

14 artificial body part

15 bend a joint

16 arthritis that affects total body and lubrication in joints

Down

1 exercises to prevent complications

2 replacement of a joint

3 surgery to insert hip prosthesis

5 turning a joint in a circle

8 partial tearing of a muscle, tendon, or ligament

9 way the body moves and keeps its balance

11 canvas belt placed around client's waist to hold onto when transferring or walking a client

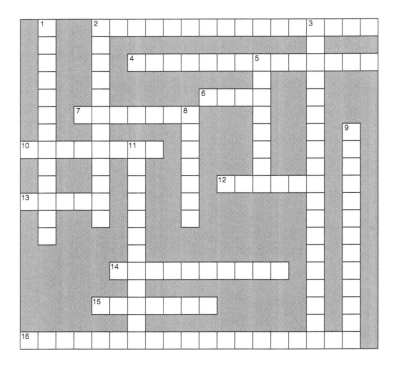

UNIT QUIZ

Short Answer/Fill in the Blanks. *Complete the following sentences with the correct word or words.*

1. The bones and muscles make up the _____ _____.

2. The shoulders and hips are _____ and _____ joints.

3. The strong muscles of the _____, _____, and _____ are the body parts meant to do heavy work.

4. A client with a fractured hip needs to avoid _____, internal and external rotation of the affected hip.

5. Total hip arthroplasty involves insertion of a hip _____.

6. Decreased activity can cause weight gain, _____, and pressure sore development.

7. When positioning a client in a side-lying position, the aide needs to check that the _____ _____ is in correct alignment.

8. List five principles of good body mechanics.

   a. _____

   b. _____

   c. _____

   d. _____

   e. _____

9. If an unsteady client starts to fall, _____ _____ the client to the floor.

10. When moving a bedridden client up in bed, use a _____.

True or False. *Answer the following statements true (T) or false (F).*

11. T   F   If the client complains of itching under the cast, the aide should blow hot air from a hair dryer into the cast.

12. T   F   Arthritis means inflammation of a muscle.

13. T   F   Home health aides need to do as much as possible for clients with musculoskeletal problems to allow clients to rest their muscles.

14. T   F   Activities are useful in helping a client relearn skills that have been lost because of illness or accident.

15. T   F   The interior of the bones produce new blood cells for the circulatory system.

16. T   F   Muscles move in response to messages from the nervous system.

17. T   F   Dangling involves placing a client's head between the knees due to nosebleed.

18. T   F   An incentive spirometer is used after surgery to encourage deep breathing and prevent pneumonia.

19. T   F   The evening is the most difficult time of day for clients with arthritis.

20. T   F   When lifting from the floor, bend your back then lift.

Matching. *Match each term with the correct definition.*

21. _____ abduction

22. _____ active range-of-motion exercises

23. _____ arthritis

24. _____ bursitis

25. _____ falls

26. _____ fracture

27. _____ gout

28. _____ rheumatoid arthritis

29. _____ osteoarthritis

30. _____ sprain

a. break in the bone

b. most common cause of injury

c. inflammation of the joints

d. inflammation of the sac between muscles and tendons

e. partial tear of a muscle, tendon, or ligament

f. wear and tear arthritis

g. arthritis that affects clients of all ages

h. arthritis due to buildup of uric acid

i. exercises performed by the client

j. move a part away from midline

Multiple Choice. *Choose the correct answer or answers.*

31. Osteoarthritis most commonly affects

   a. the hips and knees

   b. the fingers

   c. the spine

   d. small joints in the fingers, hands, and wrists

32. The greatest risk associated with osteoporosis is
    a. low back pain
    b. gradual loss of height
    c. stooped posture
    d. fractures

33. The spinal nerves are covered by the
    a. skull
    b. sternum
    c. scapula
    d. spinal column

34. Bones are joined together by tough elastic bands called
    a. ligaments
    b. tendons
    c. joints
    d. muscles

35. The most common drugs used to treat arthritis today are
    a. aspirin
    b. Tylenol
    c. anti-inflammatory medications
    d. steroids

36. Side effects of anti-inflammatory medications are
    a. black stool
    b. bloody urine
    c. ringing in the ears
    d. all of the above

37. Which of the following basic rules of body mechanics is not correct?
    a. Use the weight of your body to help push or pull an object.
    b. Keep your feet apart, to provide a good base of support.
    c. Bend from the knees when lifting.
    d. Twist your body as you work and bend to reach items.

38. While transferring Mr. Jackson from his wheelchair to bed, you need to
    a. position client with strong side toward bed
    b. place wheelchair at 45° angle
    c. lock wheels
    d. all of the above

39. Mrs. Arnez needs to be transferred using a mechanical lift. Safety concerns include
    a. Check slings, chains, and straps for frayed areas or defective hooks.
    b. Place sling with narrow piece under knees and wide piece under client's shoulder.
    c. Place sling with wide piece under knees and narrow piece under client's shoulder.
    d. Place horseshoe base at side of bed.

40. Despite cerebral palsy, 12-year-old Joseph broke his leg playing soccer and has a long leg cast. The home health aide needs to
    a. Check the cast daily for signs of roughness around the edges.
    b. Note the color of the skin at the farthest end of the cast and check for edema.
    c. Elevate his cast above the level of his heart.
    d. Don't worry about complaints of pain, as the client is taking pain medications.

UNIT 16   NERVOUS SYSTEM

LEARNING OBJECTIVES

After studying this unit, you should be able to:
- List three functions of the nervous system
- Define paraplegia, quadriplegia, and hemiplegia
- Discuss the signs of Parkinson's disease
- Discuss the disease multiple sclerosis and it's main signs and symptoms
- Discuss the disease amyotrophic lateral sclerosis and its main signs and symptoms
- Discuss epilepsy and the various types of seizures
- Explain how to care for a client having a major seizure
- Discuss the disease muscular dystrophy and its major symptoms and the age group it affects
- List ways to prevent a stroke from occurring
- List four warning signs of a stroke
- List three causes of strokes
- Discuss residual effects of a stroke
- List two types of aphasia
- Discuss the role of the aide in assisting a client recovering from a stroke
- Demonstrate the following:
  Procedure 68   Caring for a Client Having a Seizure

TERMS TO DEFINE

- amyotrophic lateral sclerosis (ALS)
- aneurysm
- aphasia
- arteriogram
- atherosclerosis
- carotid arteries
- cerebral hemorrhage
- cerebral infarction
- cerebrovascular accident (CVA)
- computed tomography (CT)
- embolus
- epilepsy
- expressive aphasia
- hemiplegia
- hemorrhage
- hypertension
- magnetic resonance imaging (MRI)
- multi-infarct dementia
- multiple sclerosis (MS)
- muscular dystrophy

- neurologist
- occupational therapist
- paraplegia
- Parkinson's disease
- plaque

- quadriplegia
- receptive aphasia
- seizure
- thrombus
- transient ischemic attack (TIA)

APPLICATION EXERCISES

Short Answer/Fill in the Blanks. *Complete the following sentences with the correct word or words.*

1. The nervous system is made up of the _____, _____ _____, and _____.

2. The five senses are _____, _____, _____, _____, and _____.

3. The master control of the nervous system is the _____.

4. Messages are relayed to the brain from _____ _____ _____ _____; the brain decides how to respond to each message.

5. Each area of the brain performs a _____ duty.

6. The spinal cord is protected by the _____ _____; if the spinal cord is damaged or diseased the spinal _____ are affected.

7. The time it takes to respond to a stimulus is called _____ time.

8. Paralysis of the lower part of the body is called _____.

9. _____ refers to paralysis of both arms and both legs.

10. Paralysis of one side of the body is called _____ and is frequently the result of a cerebrovascular accident (_____), known as a stroke.

11. Three disorders of the nervous system are:

    a. _____

    b. _____

    c. _____

12. A progressive degenerative disease characterized by shaking, fixated facial expression, shuffling gait, stiffness of limbs, and stooped posture is called _____ _____.

13. Treatment for Parkinson's disease involves _____ _____ to restore the brain's supply of dopamine with common medications such as Artane, Cogentin, and Sinemet.

14. A central nervous system disease, _____ _____ begins with episodes that last a few weeks or months separated by periods of _____, which is absence of symptoms.

15. List five symptoms seen in clients with multiple sclerosis (MS).

a. _____

b. _____

c. _____

d. _____

e. _____

16. Known as Lou Gehrig's disease, _____ _____
_____ is a gradual progressive degeneration of the nerve cells in the brain and
spinal cord that control the voluntary muscles.

17. The signs and symptoms of ALS include slow loss of _____ and coordination
in one or more limbs; muscle twitches and cramps; increasingly stiff, clumsy
_____; and difficulty with _____, speaking, or
_____. The person's mind _____ _____ while
his or her body wastes away.

18. A chronic brain disorder characterized by a sudden episode of intense electrical activity in
the brain, which results in seizure activities is called _____.

19. List the classification of seizures and the effects on the body.

a. _____

b. _____

20. Name five care activities the home health aide should perform for a client having a seizure.

a. _____

b. _____

c. _____

d. _____

e. _____

21. _____ _____ is an inherited, progressive disease caused by
lack of a key protein essential to muscle function, which causes the muscles to
_____ in size and grow _____.

22. Symptoms of muscular dystrophy are muscle _____, lack of
_____, inability to lift _____ _____
_____ _____ _____, and progressive
_____ resulting in loss of mobility.

23. Spinal cord injuries result in loss of _____ and _____ in the
body parts below the level of injury, with many clients spending the remainder of their life in
a _____.

24. Stroke is the common term for _____ _____
(_____) and is caused by a lack of _____ and nutrients to the
brain cells.

25. Interruption of blood flow to the brain may be due to:

a. _____

b. _____

c. _____

26. The most common cause of a CVA is _____.

27. Risk factors in stroke include:

    a. _____

    b. _____

    c. _____

28. Sometimes called "small strokes," _____ _____
_____ (_____) consist of a brief period of
_____, loss of _____, or a loss of _____ that
lasts minutes to hours then goes away completely.

29. TIAs are caused by a sudden but _____ decrease or stoppage of blood flow to
a part of the brain.

30. Symptoms reported by clients having a TIA include:

    a. _____

    b. _____

    c. _____

    d. _____

    e. _____

31. A health care provider who specializes in diagnosis and treatment of neurological diseases is
called a _____.

32. An _____ is a series of x-ray pictures that show the flow of blood in the
arteries, neck, and head taken after injection of intravenous (IV) dye into the artery.

33. A common form of dementia that is the result of a series of multiple strokes damaging brain
tissue is called _____ _____.

34. _____ _____ is the most common form of stroke and occurs
when a portion of the brain dies due to a blocked artery and blood is prevented from reaching
that part of the brain.

35. Bleeding into the brain, which destroys or disrupts brain tissue, is a _____
_____.

36. _____ _____ _____ is the main risk factor for
hemorrhage into the brain.

37. Signs and symptoms of cerebrovascular accident include:

    a. _____

    b. _____

    c. _____

    d. _____

    e. _____

38. Two tests performed to diagnose and assist in treatment of cerebrovascular accident are
_____ _____ _____ and _____
_____.

39. List five physical deficits resulting from CVA.

   a. _____

   b. _____

   c. _____

   d. _____

   e. _____

40. Five perceptual/cognitive deficits that may occur due to CVA include:

   a. _____

   b. _____

   c. _____

   d. _____

   e. _____

41. Personal and family problems that may occur as a result of CVA include:

   a. _____

   b. _____

   c. _____

42. The psychological effects of a stroke include _____, apathy, _____, hostility, and euphoria.

43. Aftercare of a stroke focuses on _____, with a care plan developed for each client's needs.

44. The focus of the client care plan for the stroke client is to have the client return to the _____ _____ _____ _____ as possible.

45. The home health aide needs to encourage the client to do _____ _____ _____ _____ with as little assistance as possible from others.

46. _____ is important in the rehabilitation of a client after a stroke, with the home health aide needing to walk on the client's _____ side.

47. Name five care activities the stroke client may need the assistance of the home health aide to perform.

   a. _____

   b. _____

   c. _____

   d. _____

   e. _____

48. The health care team member who will assist the stroke client in improving activities of daily living (like regaining independence in feeding) is called an _____ _____.

49. _____ is a condition in which the ability to speak is impaired and can affect the ability to talk, _____, read, or _____.

50. A client with _____ aphasia does not understand words someone else says, while a client with _____ aphasia understands words spoken but cannot express himself or herself correctly.

51. The _____ _____ will assist the client with communication problems and inform the aide of the client's type of aphasia and how to communicate more effectively.

True or False. *Answer the following statements true (T) or false (F).*

52. T   F   The nervous system can be referred to as the communication network of the body.

53. T   F   The nerve endings can be compared with electrical outlets.

54. T   F   The brain alerts other parts of the body and gives them instructions on how to respond to stimuli.

55. T   F   If the spinal cord is cut, the body could still feel the parts below the cut.

56. T   F   ALS is another name for Lou Gehrig's disease.

57. T   F   There is no cure for muscular dystrophy.

58. T   F   You should try to limit the movements of a client during a seizure.

59. T   F   Multiple sclerosis is a disease affecting the central nervous system.

60. T   F   Brain cells die when they are without oxygen for four minutes

61. T   F   Once destroyed, brain cells can be brought back to life with thrombolytic drugs.

Matching. *Match each term with the correct definition.*

62. _____   aneurysm
63. _____   brain
64. _____   CVA
65. _____   embolus
66. _____   expressive aphasia
67. _____   hemiplegia
68. _____   involuntary speech
69. _____   nerves
70. _____   nervous system
71. _____   paraplegia
72. _____   quadriplegia
73. _____   receptive aphasia
74. _____   seizure
75. _____   TIA
76. _____   thrombus

a. paralysis of one side of the body

b. stroke

c. communication center of the body

d. ballooning out of the wall of the artery

e. the control center of the nervous system

f. paralysis of both arms and legs

g. involuntary muscular contractions with loss of consciousness

h. brief period of weakness, loss of speech or feeling

i. paralysis of the lower part of the body

j. blood clot that forms inside an artery

k. part of the nervous system that receives stimuli

l. does not understand words someone else says

m. a moving blood clot

n. understands words spoken but cannot express himself or herself after CVA

o. curse words or nonsense syllables spoken by stroke client

Multiple Choice. *Choose the correct answer or answers.*

77. Medications for the client with Parkinson's disease may cause serious side effects. The home health aide should watch for and report

    a. frequent urination

    b. constipation

    c. involuntary movements, dizziness, nausea

    d. none of these

78. Parkinson's disease

    a. starts in adolescence

    b. starts in middle age

    c. involves muscle tremors and shuffling gait

    d. has episodes of seizure activity

79. Care of clients with Parkinson's disease includes

    a. regular exercise program

    b. rest periods due to fluctuating activity levels

    c. participation in support groups

    d. all of the above

80. The nervous system is composed of

    a. the lungs and heart

    b. the long bones and small bones of the leg

    c. the brain, spinal cord, and nerves

    d. none of these

81. The disease that affects only males and is a rare, inherited illness due to a lack of a key protein essential to muscle function is called

    a. muscular dystrophy

    b. multiple sclerosis

    c. epilepsy

    d. amyotrophic lateral sclerosis

82. If the spinal cord is damaged below the waist, the client will be

    a. hemiplegic

    b. paraplegic

    c. quadriplegic

    d. none of the above

83. The client who broke his neck and upper spine in a diving accident would be

    a. hemiplegic

    b. paraplegic

    c. quadriplegic

    d. none of the above

84. Loss of movement of one side of the body seen-post CVA would result in the client being

    a. hemiplegic

    b. paraplegic

    c. quadriplegic

    d. none of the above

85. Clients with multiple sclerosis often have a wide variety of symptoms including

    a. poor coordination of muscle movements with numbness or tingling sensations

    b. blurred or double vision

    c. problems with bowel and bladder control

    d. all of the above

86. Most clients with multiple sclerosis

    a. live productive lives

    b. may need adaptive devices such as cane or walker

    c. have increasing difficulty swallowing

    d. suffer from a lack of energy and fatigue easily

87. The symptoms of amyotrophic lateral sclerosis include all but
    a. onset of gradual weakness in one upper extremity then the next
    b. muscle twitches and cramps with increasingly stiff gait
    c. difficulty with swallowing, speaking, and breathing, with complete paralysis ensuing
    d. progressive decline in mental function resulting in dementia

88. A chronic brain disorder characterized by sudden electrical impulses, which results in seizure activity is called
    a. muscular dystrophy   c. epilepsy
    b. multiple sclerosis   d. amyotrophic lateral sclerosis

89. Clients who have periods of just staring into space, smacking their lips, or twitching of an arm may be experiencing
    a. grand mal seizure   c. loss of consciousness
    b. epileptic fit   d. partial seizure

90. Suddenly you see a person cry out, fall to the ground, and become unconscious. Their body becomes stiff and there is shaking of the entire body with foaming at the mouth. This is an example of a
    a. grand mal seizure   c. loss of consciousness
    b. epileptic fit   d. partial seizure

91. During a seizure, the home health aide should
    a. roll the client to the side   c. loosen clothing
    b. not limit the movements of the client d. all of the above

92. It is important for a client with epilepsy to
    a. get plenty of exercise with rest periods c. take medications as prescribed
    b. wear a Medic Alert bracelet or necklace   d. drink six to eight glasses of water a day

93. Most spinal cord injures are the result of
    a. traffic or industrial accidents   c. sports injuries
    b. gunshot wounds   d. all of the above

94. Spinal cord injury involves
    a. loss of sensation   c. aphasia or loss of speech
    b. loss of function of body part   d. decline in mental function
       below injury

95. Approximately 66% of strokes that occur yearly are in individuals
    a. over age 65   c. who are Caucasian
    b. of African American and   d. under age 65
       Hispanic descent

96. The symptoms of cerebrovascular accident include
    a. low blood pressure   c. vision disturbances and language
                                                  problems
    b. paralysis of limbs   d. mental confusion

97. Controllable risk factors for cerebrovascular accident include all but
    a. atherosclerosis
    b. high cholesterol
    c. obesity
    d. excess alcohol intake

98. Most transient ischemic attacks (TIAs) are caused by
    a. arteriosclerosis
    b. platelet clumping
    c. excess alcohol intake
    d. cerebral hemorrhage

99. The treatment of TIA may involve
    a. carotid endarterectomy surgery
    b. cholesterol reduction
    c. medications that reduce blood clotting
    d. anti-inflammatory medications

100. Bleeding into the brain which destroys or disrupts brain tissue is called
    a. cerebral infarction
    b. cerebral hemorrhage
    c. cerebrovascular accident
    d. cerebral ischemia

101. The main risk factor for cerebral hemorrhage is
    a. high blood pressure
    b. atherosclerosis
    c. obesity
    d. excess alcohol intake

102. The client who suffers a stroke usually has all but
    a. loses consciousness
    b. becomes incontinent of urine or feces
    c. labored or difficult breathing
    d. diminished mental function

103. Clients with communication problems may use the following to improve communication
    a. adaptive utensils
    b. ambulatory aids such as cane or walker
    c. communication board
    d. speech therapy exercises

Documentation Exercises. *Read the following descriptions and provide documentation for each scenario.*

104. You are caring for a client who has had a stroke. While you are bathing her, she starts to have a seizure. She convulses for two minutes. You quickly turn her to her side and gently hold her on the bed until she stops convulsing. After the seizure has stopped, she goes to sleep. You notice she has wet the bed. You call and report this to your nurse. How would you document this?

105. When you arrive at your client's home, you find him sitting on the couch waiting for you. He wants to go to the grocery store and shop. You have been given specific instructions to bathe him and prepare a meal. You know the physical therapist is due to work with him in about an hour. You know that he dislikes his therapy treatments. How would you handle this situation and how would you document it?

Label the Diagram

106. Label the parts of the nervous system in the diagram; refer to Figure 16–1.

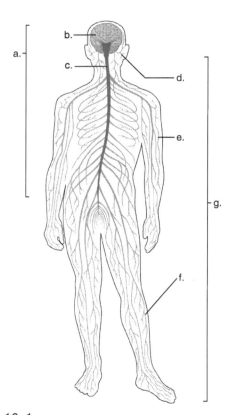

a. _____

b. _____

c. _____

d. _____

e. _____

f. _____

g. _____

Figure 16–1

PRACTICE SITUATIONS

Case 1

You have been assigned to a new client, Mr. Shoji. He is a 45-year-old man who has had his left lower leg amputated. Part of your assignment is to help attach the prosthesis and help him into the chair. When you are ready to help him, he tells you that he has never attached the prosthesis and expects that you will take care of it.

Questions

1. What can you do?
2. How can you perform your assignment and not let him know that you have never done this before?
3. Can you think of anything you can say to him that will help?

Case 2

You are assigned to Mrs. Suzy who had a cerebrovascular accident two months ago. She is impulsive and attempts to do things she is not yet ready for. Today, while you reached for her clean clothes, she decided to get into her wheelchair herself. You caught her as she slid out of the wheelchair.

Questions

1. What should you do now?
2. What should you report?
3. Who do you notify?
4. What can you do to avoid this in the future?

CROSSWORD PUZZLE

Across

3 fatty deposits in the arteries

4 central nervous system disease

5 hardening of the arteries

9 ability to speak is impaired

11 blood clot that forms inside an artery

13 interruption of blood flow to the brain

14 paralysis of one side of the body

Down

1 brief period of weakness and loss of speech or feeling

2 blood vessel in the neck supplying blood to brain

6 episodes of intense electrical activity in the brain

7 paralysis of both arms and both legs

8 ballooning out of the wall of the artery

10 a moving blood clot

12 health care provider who cares for client with neuromuscular problems

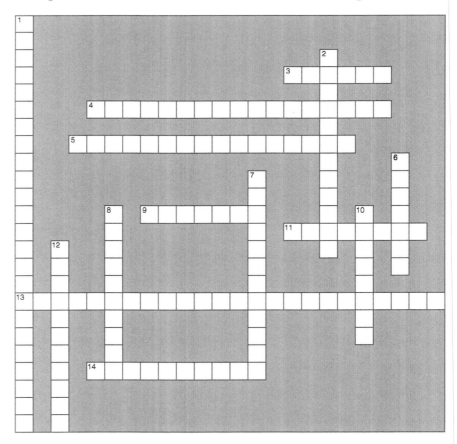

UNIT QUIZ

Short Answer/Fill in the Blanks. *Complete the following sentences with the correct word or words.*

1. The communication center that sends messages to all parts of the body is the

   _____ _____.

2. The _____ is the master control or switch of the nervous system.

3. _____ are relayed to the brain from all parts of the body with the brain deciding how to respond to each message/stimulus sent by the _____.

4. All the major nerves of the body are bound together in the _____ _____ and lead to the brain.

5. If the spinal cord is cut or damaged, the _____ below the cut no longer send messages up to the brain; the parts of the body below the cut no longer feel _____, and the muscles don't _____.

6. The nerve _____ in the body are usually ready to receive stimuli and send messages to the brain, with the entire process taking place in an instant.

7. The time it takes to respond to a stimulus is known as the _____ _____, with the time often slowing down as the body ages.

8. List five nervous system disorders.

   a. _____

   b. _____

   c. _____

   d. _____

   e. _____

9. Brain cells die when they are without oxygen for _____ minutes.

10. Brain cells can _____ by taking over duties of other cells when brain damage has occurred.

True of False. *Answer the following statements true (T) or false (F).*

11. T   F   A CT scan will show if there has been brain damage or injury.

12. T   F   Quadriplegia is paralysis of one side of the body.

13. T   F   To reach the brain, messages travel through the spinal cord.

14. T   F   Once brain cell death occurs, there is no chance of new cells forming.

15. T   F   Stroke is always caused by high blood pressure.

Matching. *Match each term with the correct definition.*

16. _____   aneurysm

17. _____   atherosclerosis

18. _____   arteriogram

19. _____   embolus

20. _____   expressive aphasia

21. _____   hemiplegia

22. _____   quadriplegia

23. _____   paraplegia

24. _____   receptive aphasia

25. _____   thrombus

a. fatty deposits in the arteries

b. hardening of the arteries

c. ballooning out of the wall of the artery

d. blood clot that forms inside an artery

e. paralysis of one side of the body

f. x-ray test with IV dye that shows the flow of blood in the arteries, neck, and head

g. paralysis of both arms and both legs

h. inability to express oneself after CVA

i. paralysis of the lower part of the body

j. does not understand words someone else says

Multiple Choice. *Choose the correct answer or answers.*

26. All of the following are part of the nervous system except

    a. brain

    b. muscles

    c. spinal cord

    d. nerves

27. Quadriplegia refers to paralysis of

    a. one arm and one leg

    b. both arms

    c. both legs

    d. both arms and both legs

28. Common symptoms of nervous system disorders include

    a. shakiness in the extremities (tremors)

    b. difficulty walking

    c. mental changes

    d. all of the above

29. Mr. White has been battling Parkinson's disease for seven years. He ambulates with a quad cane. Signs you may observe include

    a. shuffling walking pattern

    b. shakiness of the body at rest

    c. stooped posture

    d. none of the above

30. A care plan for Mr. White may include

    a. cutting food into small pieces

    b. preparing a well-balanced, nutritious meal

    c. encouraging rest periods between activities

    d. encouraging client to perform range-of-motion (ROM) exercises

31. Mr. Simmons has been slowly losing strength in his left arm and now the right is affected. He has muscle twitches and cramps and increasingly stiff, clumsy gait. Swallowing meat is difficult at times. The doctor told him he has Lou Gehrig's disease, known as

    a. muscular dystrophy

    b. multiple sclerosis

    c. epilepsy

    d. amyotrophic lateral sclerosis

32. Since the age of 28, Mrs. O'Hara has had problems with poor coordination of muscle movements, numbness, and tingling in her legs. In her 40s, she had double vision and partial blindness. By age 50, she had gone into remission and was able to work for 10 years. Now at age 65, she has a reoccurrence of weakness in her legs, fatigues easily, and uses a cane. Last week she tripped over a rug and fell. She is taking Prednisone medication to treat her illness. She bruises very easily and has skin tears on her arms. Her diagnosis is

    a. muscular dystrophy   c. epilepsy

    b. multiple sclerosis   d. amyotrophic lateral sclerosis

33. Mrs. O'Hara's care plan includes

    a. recommending wheelchair ambulation

    b. padding sharp edges of furniture and doorways

    c. using a shower chair and assistance with bathing

    d. encouraging client to remove scatter rugs from her home

34. Sixteen-year-old Jonathan has been using a walker for 10 years. His legs are so weak that he now uses a wheelchair. Unable to lift his arms over his head, he requires assistance getting dressed. Jonathan's medical condition is called

    a. muscular dystrophy   c. epilepsy

    b. multiple sclerosis   d. amyotrophic lateral sclerosis

35. Mr. Fernandez is visiting his elderly mother who you are assisting when he suddenly collapses to the floor, becomes unconscious, and then his entire body begins shaking uncontrollably. You realize he is having a seizure. What should you do next?

    a. Call 911.

    b. Remove any surrounding furniture or objects to avoid injury.

    c. Turn his head to the side to prevent aspirating secretions and biting the tongue.

    d. All of the above

36. Mr. Fernandez was diagnosed with

    a. muscular dystrophy   c. epilepsy

    b. multiple sclerosis   d. amyotrophic lateral sclerosis

37. Two months ago, Mr. Dali had a cerebrovascular accident due to an aneurysm. The most important aspect of his care at home focuses on

    a. rehabilitation   c. diet therapy

    b. home adaptation   d. all of the above

38. Risk factors in stroke include

    a. hypertension   c. cancer

    b. atherosclerosis   d. diabetes

39. Mr. Dali has left-sided weakness. When walking with the client, the home health aide should

    a. walk in front of the client

    b. walk behind the client

    c. walk beside the client on his strong side

    d. walk beside the client on his weak side

40. Mr. Dali is easily frustrated with dressing himself due to fumbling with buttons. The home health aide should

    a. take over the task to ease the client's frustration

    b. offer encouragement to the client

    c. do not rush client through his routine

    d. discuss with occupational therapist the client's difficulties and inquire about the use of assistive devices

UNIT 17   CIRCULATORY SYSTEM

LEARNING OBJECTIVES

After studying this unit, you should be able to:
- Name the main function of the heart
- Name three types of blood vessels
- List at least six risk factors for heart problems
- Describe an angina attack and when it usually occurs
- Explain the effect of nitroglycerin on the blood vessels
- Describe the signs and symptoms of a myocardial infarction
- Describe congestive heart failure and how it is treated
- List three blood disorders
- List three symptoms of arterial insufficiency
- Describe three ways the aide can assist in the care of a client with thrombophlebitis
- Demonstrate the following:
  Procedure 69   Applying Elasticized Stockings

TERMS TO DEFINE

- activities of daily living (ADL)
- anemia
- angina pectoris
- angiogram
- angioplasty
- anticoagulants
- arterial insufficiency
- arteriosclerosis
- artery
- cardiac arrest
- catheterization
- collateral circulation
- congestive heart failure
- cyanosis
- echocardiogram
- edema
- electrocardiogram
- gangrene
- hemophilia
- hypotension
- intermittent claudication
- iron deficiency anemia
- ischemia
- leukemia
- myocardial infarction
- myocardium
- nitroglycerin
- pernicious anemia
- phlebitis
- pulmonary embolus

■ sickle cell anemia

■ thrombophlebitis

■ sublingually

■ venous insufficiency

APPLICATION EXERCISES

Short Answer/Fill in the Blanks. *Complete the following sentences with the correct word or words.*

1. The organ that supplies power to the body system is the _____.

2. The purpose of the heart is to _____ _____
   _____ _____ _____.

3. There are _____ chambers in the hollow muscular organ that is the heart: the right and left _____ and the right and left _____.

4. The _____ atrium receives oxygen-poor blood from the tissues.

5. The _____ ventricle pumps the blood to the lungs, where it picks up _____, while blood is pumped out to all parts of the body through the _____ ventricle.

6. There are three kinds of blood vessels:

   a. _____

   b. _____

   c. _____

7. Blood is carried away from the heart to the body's cells in blood vessels called _____.

8. Tiny blood vessels between the arteries and the veins are called _____.

9. The veins carry blood back to the _____.

10. The heart _____, meaning squeezes together and _____, relaxes.

11. The pulse measured at the wrist is the expansion of the _____ _____.

12. Arterial blood is _____ _____ in color; this is due to its oxygen content.

13. Venous blood is a darker red because of its low _____ content.

14. Age-related changes that affect the circulatory system include:

    a. _____

    b. _____

    c. _____

15. Six risk factors for cardiovascular disease include:

    a. _____

    b. _____

    c. _____

    d. _____

    e. _____

    f. _____

16. The number one cause of death in the United States is _____ _____.

17. If an infant is born with a heart defect, it is called a _____ heart problem.

18. The majority of individuals who survive after a heart attack will need medical care and assistance with _____ _____ _____ _____.

19. Disorders of the heart and circulatory system force people to change their _____.

20. Many people become very _____ when they are told they have heart disease.

21. Some heart conditions require that clients _____ their activity.

22. _____ pectoris is a symptom of a condition called myocardial ischemia, which occurs when the heart muscle, or _____ does not get an adequate supply of _____ and _____ to do its work.

23. A person having an episode of angina pectoris will become _____ and _____ with the body stiffening; the blood pressure will _____; the client will then become flushed and _____ heavily. Clients may have a mild pain that radiates from the chest to the _____ arm and up to the neck or a feeling of fullness, _____, aching, _____, _____, or painful feeling in the chest, upper back, or jaw. Immediate treatment for angina is physical _____.

24. A common emergency medication for angina is _____. It can be taken _____ (under the tongue), in spray form, or in the form of a patch placed on the skin. The home health aide may have to assist the client in placing the new patch on the skin. Make sure that _____ patches are removed and the skin cleansed thoroughly with soap and water before a _____ patch is applied. This is to prevent a buildup effect from residual nitroglycerin. Application sites should be alternated daily to prevent _____ _____.

25. Nitroglycerin opens the _____ _____ to increase _____ _____. The effect of the drug occurs within _____ to _____ minutes with angina usually relieved in _____ to _____ minutes. If the client does not get relief from pain with three tablets/sprays taken over a time span of 15 minutes, _____ _____ is required with the home health aide encouraged to call 911.

26. Nitroglycerin loses its _____ and effectiveness over time and needs to be kept in the original bottle and out of light to maintain its potency. The home health aide should check the _____ _____.

27. List five things clients with angina can do to maintain health.

   a. _____

   b. _____

   c. _____

   d. _____

   e. _____

28. A myocardial infarction is more commonly known as a _____ _____; a condition when the blood vessel of the _____ _____ closes or is blocked by a blood clot, which causes _____ _____ to the heart muscle.

29. Smaller vessels sometimes take over the work of the blocked _____. This is referred to as collateral circulation.

30. List five symptoms of a heart attack.

   a. _____

   b. _____

   c. _____

   d. _____

   e. _____

31. Tests used to diagnose a myocardial infarction include _____, test done that can determine how the heart is pumping and what areas are not pumping; exercise stress test; and an _____, recording of heart electrical activity.

32. Emergency care is needed for the client after a heart attack as the person may go into _____ and _____.

33. During a cardiac catheterization, a catheter tube is passed into a vein or artery then through the heart to detect _____.

34. In coronary _____ procedure, a health care provider inserts a catheter with a balloon at the end of it, threaded through the coronary arteries and when the blockage is located, the balloon is inflated and the plaque or obstruction is flattened and the artery is reopened.

35. A common operation performed to restore heart muscle blood circulation is called coronary artery bypass grafting, or _____.

36. _____ are drugs that thin the blood and slow the clotting time. The home health aide needs to observe the client who is taking this medication for signs of bleeding. Two signs the aide needs to watch for are _____ _____ and _____ _____; if they occur, the aide needs to _____ _____ _____ _____.

37. If a person's heart stops beating it is called _____ _____.

38. A condition in which the heart does not pump effectively is called _____ _____ _____.

39. Symptoms of congestive heart failure include:

   a. _____

   b. _____

   c. _____

   d. _____

   e. _____

40. Treatment of congestive heart failure includes _____, which slows and strengthens the heartbeat, and a _____, which reduces fluid accumulation in the body.

41. Three things the home health aide taking care of the client with congestive heart failure needs to remember are:

   a. _____

   b. _____

   c. _____

42. A condition in which the arteries become hard and lose their elasticity is _____. This is caused by the buildup of _____ _____ on the inside walls of the blood vessels.

43. Risk factors for arteriosclerosis are people who _____, and have _____ _____ and high blood pressure.

44. _____ _____ is due to damage of the veins that return blood to the heart.

45. If the client complains of aching in the legs, has edema of the legs, and the legs are discolored, the client could be experiencing venous insufficiency. The aide needs to report these complaints to the _____.

46. Thrombophlebitis is a serious condition and occurs when the vein becomes inflamed and a clot forms. If the client has tenderness, warmth, or _____ in the calf of the leg, the aide should report it _____ to the nurse.

47. A life-threatening condition that is a complication of thrombophlebitis is _____ _____.

48. Arterial insufficiency is a condition that is caused by narrowing of the _____ that supply blood to the lower extremities. When the client walks or exercises, the leg muscles may become _____ in the calf or thigh; this is called _____ _____, with the pain subsiding after a few minutes of rest.

49. The purpose of applying elasticized stockings is

   a. _____

   b. _____

   c. _____

50. Signs of compete obstruction include severe _____, pallor, absence of _____ in lower leg, numbness, paralysis, and _____ of the limb.

51. Death of the body tissue caused by lack of adequate blood supply is called _____. Signs are fever, pain, _____ _____ _____ _____, and unpleasant odor.

52. List four main parts of blood.

   a. _____

   b. _____

   c. _____

   d. _____

53. Five disorders of the blood include:

   a. _____

   b. _____

   c. _____

   d. _____

   e. _____

54. When there is not enough blood cells due to excessive blood loss, malformation of blood cells, or lack of essential nutrients _____ occurs.

55. The most common nutrient deficiency in the world is _____ _____. Treatment includes taking an _____ _____ or eating iron-rich foods such as _____ _____, beans, _____ _____ _____, and fortified breads and cereals.

56. _____ _____ is caused by the body's inability to produce the intrinsic factor, vitamin B_{12} resulting in damage to red blood cells and the nervous system.

57. The inherited disease _____ _____ _____ is caused by red blood cells that are _____ shaped. The cells are unable to carry enough oxygen in them, causing anemia.

58. A condition where there are too many immature white blood cells is called _____, also called cancer of the blood. Clients are very prone to _____ and need to avoid crowds of persons and those with _____.

59. A hereditary disease characterized by spontaneous bleeding due to a lack of a clotting factor in the blood is called _____.

True or False. *Answer the following statements true (T) or false (F).*

60. T   F   Men have a greater risk of having a heart attack than premenopausal women.

61. T   F   As people grow older, they have less chance of having a heart attack.

62. T   F   Individuals whose parents had heart problems will have a greater chance of having heart disease themselves.

63. T   F   People with high cholesterol levels in their blood have less chance of heart disease.

64. T   F   As stress increases in a person's life, so does the risk of heart attack.

65. T   F   People who are overweight, smoke, or have diabetes are at risk for heart disease.

66. T   F   Increasing exercise is a good way to increase the risk of heart attack.

67. T   F   The home health aide is very important in the care of the client who has heart disease.

68. T   F   The effects of nitroglycerin generally occur within two to three hours.

69. T   F   A Coronary Artery Bypass Graph (CABG) is an operation commonly performed on the heart for blocked coronary vessels.

Matching. *Match each term with the correct definition.*

70. _____ angina pectoris

71. _____ arterial insufficiency

72. _____ arteriosclerosis

73. _____ cardiac arrest

74. _____ collateral circulation

75. _____ congestive heart failure

76. _____ hemophilia

77. _____ hypotension

78. _____ pulmonary embolus

a. hardening of the arteries

b. low blood pressure

c. small heart vessels take over work of blocked arteries

d. hereditary disease with lack of clotting factor

e. heart muscle receives inadequate oxygenation, causing pain

f. blood clot in the lung

g. heart stops beating

h. narrowing of lower leg veins

i. ineffective heart pumping

Multiple Choice. *Choose the correct answer or answers.*

79. The circulatory system is made up of the
    a. heart, arteries, veins, capillaries
    b. heart, arteries, sinuses, veins
    c. heart, lungs, veins, capillaries
    d. heart, lungs, arteries, capillaries

80. Venous blood is dark red due to
    a. being low in oxygen
    b. client having anemia
    c. being enriched with oxygen
    d. passage through the capillaries

81. In order for blood to be oxygen enriched, blood needs to travel through
    a. pulmonary arteries
    b. pulmonary veins
    c. capillary beds
    d. vena cava

82. Signs of side effects of anticoagulants include
    a. bleeding from the gums
    b. bruises on the extremities
    c. tarry stools
    d. all of these

83. Death of body tissue brought on by lack of adequate blood supply to the area is called
    a. thrombosis
    b. thrombophlebitis
    c. anemia
    d. gangrene

84. The home health aide caring for the client with a blood clot in the leg should encourage the client to
    a. ambulate with a walker
    b. walk with the cane on the weaker side
    c. use crutches
    d. remain in bed

85. While caring for a client who needs elastic stockings applied, the home health aide should
    a. ask the client to sit in a chair while the aide applies the stockings
    b. apply the stockings while the client is lying down
    c. reapply the stockings each day
    d. none of these

86. A client experiencing shortness of breath, cyanotic skin and nails, and retention of fluid in the legs has signs of

    a. angina

    b. congestive heart failure

    c. pernicious anemia

    d. venous insufficiency

87. When caring for a client with congestive heart failure, the home health aide can best assist the client by

    a. reminding the client to take prescribed medications

    b. preparing a diet low in sodium and fat and high in bulk

    c. helping balance exercise with rest periods

    d. all of the above

88. Chronic aching in the legs, edema, and discoloration of the lower extremities are signs and symptoms of

    a. angina

    b. congestive heart failure

    c. pernicious anemia

    d. venous insufficiency

Documentation Exercises. *Read the following descriptions and provide documentation for each scenario.*

89. Your client has recently been discharged from the hospital. She had a heart attack. Her health care provider ordered her to start mild exercising. You have been told to walk her around the apartment twice during your time with her. When you approach her with the walker, she becomes very upset and states, "My health care provider is trying to kill me. I know if I walk around this room, I will have another heart attack and die." What can you do to help calm her down? Document this information.

90. Mrs. Kee is your second client of the day. She has a diagnosis of angina. You are running about 20 minutes later than usual. When you arrive, she is agitated. She grasps her chest and tells you she has been having chest pain all morning. You inquire if she took her nitroglycerin. She says no, so you get the medication container and Mrs. Kee takes a sublingual tablet. After a short time, she calms down and allows you to assist with her bath. Document this information.

Label the Diagram.

91. Label the parts of the cardiovascular system; refer to Figure 17–1.

a. _____

b. _____

c. _____

d. _____

e. _____

f. _____

92. Label the parts of the circulatory system; refer to Figure 17–2.

a. _____

b. _____

c. _____

d. _____

e. _____

f. _____

g. _____

h. _____

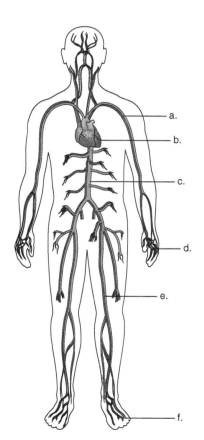

Figure 17–1

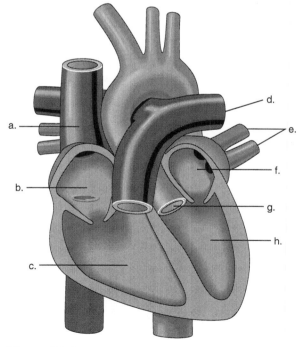

Figure 17–2

PRACTICE SITUATIONS

Case 1

Mrs. Jacinto has been assigned to you. She has recently had a heart attack. She is a very busy lady. She has several children and grandchildren. Part of her care includes rest, taking it easy, and no stress. She is having a difficult time complying with this. In fact, when you arrive, you find her in the kitchen cleaning.

Questions

1. How are you going to help your client take it easy?

2. What can you tell her?

3. Can you think of any ways to help her get her needed rest?

Case 2

Mr. Nature is on blood thinning medications. You have been instructed to watch for bleeding when you care for him. You notice that when he brushes his teeth, there is a small amount of bleeding in the sink.

Questions

1. Where else would you expect to see bleeding if he is getting too many blood thinners?

2. What should you tell the client?

3. Do you need to contact the nurse?

CROSSWORD PUZZLE

Across

1 heart attack

6 blood vessel that carries blood back to heart

7 bluish tinged skin and nails

9 blood vessel that carries blood away from heart

12 born with a health condition

13 retention of fluid

14 medication used for angina

Down

1 heart muscle

2 condition of ineffective heart pumping

3 procedure done to clear a blockage in the heart

4 vein inflammation with clot formation

5 drugs that reduce blood clotting

8 not enough red blood cells

10 hardening of the arteries

11 high blood pressure

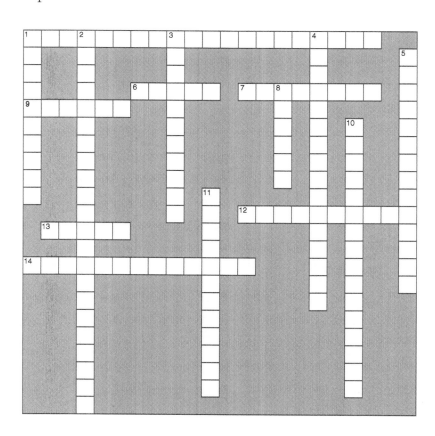

UNIT QUIZ

Short Answer/Fill in the Blanks. *Complete the following sentences with the correct word or words.*

1. As the heart _____ (squeezes together) and _____ (relaxes), it pushes blood into the arteries.

2. The three kinds of blood vessels are:

   a. _____

   b. _____

   c. _____

3. Age-related changes affecting the cardiovascular system include the heart muscle fibers becoming _____ and thick, the _____ of the heart stiffen, and the blood vessels become _____ _____.

4. The main function of the _____ is to pump blood throughout the body.

5. A mild pain in the chest lasting a few seconds, pale, ashen appearance, and body stiffness are signs of _____.

6. The medication used for angina attacks, which opens the blood vessels is called _____.

7. Two tests used to diagnose angina pectoris include _____ and _____.

8. The medical term for a heart attack or coronary is _____ _____, which is a condition in which a blood vessel of the heart muscle closes or is blocked by a blood clot.

9. List five symptoms of a heart attack.

   a. _____

   b. _____

   c. _____

   d. _____

   e. _____

10. Complications of myocardial infarction include _____ and _____.

11. Test done to detect amount of heart damage after a heart attack is cardiac _____.

12. Drugs that reduce the ability of the blood to clot are called _____, and are commonly used after a heart attack.

13. Three concerns regarding anticoagulant use include:

   a. _____

   b. _____

   c. _____

14. A blood clot traveling from the legs to the lungs causes symptoms of _____ and severe breathing problems, even _____ _____, and is known as _____ _____.

15. Cardiac arrest means that a person's heart has _____ _____.

16. Inability of the heart to pump effectively leads to a condition called _____ _____ _____.

17. Signs and symptoms of congestive heart failure include a cough, shortness of breath (_____), bluish tinged nails (_____), retention of fluid (_____), and frothy pink sputum may accumulate in the lung causing _____.

18. The home health aide must _____ apply heat to a client's cold feet if the client has arteriosclerosis; instead the client should be offered another pair of _____.

19. Venous insufficiency is due to damage of the _____ that return blood to the heart. Symptoms include chronic aching, _____, and _____ of the lower extremities.

20. Home health aides often assist with simple wound care for clients with venous insufficiency, as they are prone to _____ _____ due to lack of oxygen available to the tissues.

21. _____ occurs when the veins in the lower extremities become inflamed and a _____ _____ forms.

22. The home health aide needs to report these symptoms of thrombophlebitis to the nurse the same day noted: tenderness, _____, warmth over the vein, and _____ in the calf.

23. A serious life-threatening complication of thrombophlebitis is _____ _____, which occurs when a blood clot has broken away and traveled to the lungs.

24. Clients may need assistance applying anti-embolism stockings known as _____ or Ace wraps; the purpose of which is to:

   a. _____

   b. _____

   c. _____

True or False. *Answer the following statements true (T) or false (F).*

25. T   F   A cardiac arrest is very serious, with death occurring if CPR and resuscitation attempts fail.

26. T   F   Congestive heart failure is a heart condition that can cause swelling of the legs and feet, or fluid in the lungs.

27. T   F   Brain cells die when they do not receive oxygen for more than four minutes.

28. T   F   Inflammation of the lining of the vein is called angina.

29. T   F   Sickle cell anemia is a hereditary condition seen in African Americans and occurs when the red blood cells become sickle shaped and unable to carry oxygen.

30. T   F   A condition in which there are too many red blood cells produced by the body is called leukemia.

31. T   F   Anemia occurs when there are not enough red blood cells.

32. T   F   Only diabetics are at risk for developing gangrene.

33. T   F   Hemophilia is a hereditary disease with clients prone to spontaneous hemorrhages due to deficiency in clotting factor in the blood.

34. T   F   Clients with iron deficiency anemia are encouraged to avoid red meats, dark green leafy vegetables, beans, and fortified cereals.

Matching. *Match each term with the correct definition.*

35. ____   anemia
36. ____   aneurysm
37. ____   arteriogram
38. ____   artery
39. ____   atherosclerosis
40. ____   embolus
41. ____   ischemia
42. ____   myocardium
43. ____   thrombus
44. ____   vein

a. a blood clot that forms inside an artery
b. insufficient red blood cells
c. x-rays of blood flow in arteries
d. a moving blood clot
e. hardening of the artery
f. ballooning out of the wall of an artery
g. condition in which a portion of the heart dies
h. blood vessel carries blood away from heart
i. blood vessel carries blood back to heart
j. heart muscle

Multiple Choice. *Choose the correct answer or answers.*

45. It takes how many minutes for blood to leave the heart, travel through the arteries, capillaries, and veins and return to the heart

   a. 1 minute
   b. 4 minutes
   c.   10 minutes
   d.   60 minutes

46. The number one killer of individuals in the United States is

   a. cancer
   b. domestic abuse
   c.   vehicular accidents
   d.   cardiovascular disease

47. A major risk factor in heart disease is

   a. heredity
   b. cigarette smoking
   c. high blood pressure
   d.   high cholesterol levels
   e.   all of these

48. The home health aide's care plan for clients with cardiovascular disease focuses on assisting clients with

   a. activities of daily living
   b. meal preparation
   c.   light housekeeping
   d.   medication management

49. The function of blood within the body includes

   a. supplies cells of body with food and oxygen
   b. carries waste products to specific organs that remove the waste products from the body
   c. fights germs that enter the body
   d. all of the above

50. Mr. Le, who is 53, had severe chest pain and went to the hospital where his health care provider diagnosed a myocardial infarction. Complete cardiac workup including coronary angiography revealed he had a blocked coronary artery, and a CABG procedure was performed. After spending time in the local hospital's skilled nursing unit he is now home. His daughter Rose arrives for a visit and asks you what happened to her dad. How do you explain this in laymen's terms?

    a. "Your dad had a heart attack. His health care providers performed tests including cardiac catheterization where they looked inside the brain to see how the blood vessels performed and found a blockage. Surgery was performed to improve blood flow. He spent time recovering and getting stronger in the hospital's skilled nursing unit. Now home, he is receiving nursing and home health aide care."

    b. "Your dad had a heart attack. His health care providers performed tests including cardiac catheterization where they looked inside the heart's coronary arteries to see if there was a blockage, which they found. They then performed surgery to improve blood flow. He spent time recovering and getting stronger in the hospital's skilled nursing unit. Now home, he is receiving nursing and home health aide care, which I am providing."

    c. "Your dad had a heart attack. His health care providers performed tests including cardiac catheterization where they looked inside the arteries of the legs to see how the blood vessels were and found a blockage. They then performed surgery to improve blood flow by inserting medication into the legs. He spent time recovering and getting stronger in the hospital's skilled nursing unit. Now home, he is receiving nursing and home health aide care."

    d. "Your dad had a heart attack. His health care providers performed several tests including cardiac angioplasty and found a blockage. They then performed surgery to improve blood flow. He spent time recovering and getting stronger in the hospital's rehabilitation unit and is now receiving home care."

51. Rose asks you what she can do to help her father and wants details of his condition, asking you many detailed questions. What advice can you offer her?

    a. Doctors have prescribed a diet low in fat and cholesterol.

    b. Mr. Le has several new medications, which he is reminded to take from the med box.

    c. The care plan includes encouraging mild exercise followed by a rest period.

    d. Mr. Le's nurse can best advise you about the details of his condition. You show the daughter the agency phone number located on the refrigerator door.

    e. All of the above.

52. Since being hospitalized the first time one year ago with congestive heart failure, Mrs. Ash has had three more hospitalizations. She is now enrolled in your agency's congestive heart failure program. You arrive for your visit to find that her son has brought the client her favorite meal of fried catfish, french fries, and coleslaw. Mrs. Ash shows you her ankles, which are puffy, and says she couldn't rest on her sofa due to shortness of breath. You review the care plan with the client and her son, which includes

    a. having a diet high in fat, cholesterol, and sodium

    b. having a diet low in fat, cholesterol, and sodium

    c. checking her weight daily and calling the health care provider if there is more than a 2-pound gain in 24 hours or 5 pounds in one week

    d. recommending that she sit in a recliner or high-back chair with feet elevated on a footstool to ease breathing

53. You check Mrs. Ash's pillbox and note that she has missed two morning doses of medications in the past week. What should you do?

    a. Ask the client why she skipped the medications.

    b. Remind the client that the diuretic (water pill) is in the morning container and it is important to prevent fluid accumulation in her heart.

    c. Do nothing, as it is the nurse's job to monitor medication compliance.

    d. Notify the nurse about the skipped medications.

54. Mr. Johnson, an African American client, has been receiving home care due to a mild CVA. His past medical history includes diabetes and peripheral vascular disease. His wife has been bathing him, but she was just hospitalized. A home health aide was just added to his care plan. Upon removing his socks, you notice his right little toe is dark and hard with a foul odor. You suspect that he has

    a. athlete's foot infection

    b. elevated blood sugar

    c. cut his toenails too short

    d. gangrene

55. What should you do next for Mr. Johnson?

    a. Wash the foot with warm soapy water and rinse well, then apply a clean sock.

    b. Wash the foot with warm soapy water and rinse well, apply a dry, sterile dressing, then apply a clean sock.

    c. Call 911 and send the client to the emergency room.

    d. Notify the nurse about the foot problems.

56. Mrs. Hall has frequent angina episodes. She keeps her bottle of nitroglycerin next to her chair in the living room. Today, upon arriving at the home, you see that the cap is off the bottle and two pills are sitting next to the bottle. Mrs. Hall states that she had several episodes of chest pain starting on Friday, and the pills didn't seem to work as well as before, so it was just easier to leave the top off. What can you do next to help this client?

    a. Check the expiration date to see if the medication expired, which it had.

    b. Assist the client in having the prescription refilled at the pharmacy.

    c. Remind the client that medication needs to be kept in the original container with cap securely on to prevent losing its potency.

    d. Do nothing, as it is not in your job description.

57. Mrs. Hall admits that her eyesight is failing and she cannot see the medication labels properly, so she just takes the pills by color. What should you do with this information?

    a. Offer to read the prescription bottles to the client.

    b. Pour the medications into her med box yourself.

    c. Call her daughter and encourage an eye exam.

    d. Notify the nurse or your case manager.

58. Just diagnosed with iron deficiency anemia, Mrs. Marchucci fatigues easily and complains of being too tired to cook. Her care plan includes assisting her into the tub and preparing lunch and a snack. Which of the following would be appropriate meal choices to help increase her iron content?

    a. grilled cheese sandwich on white bread, tomato soup, small salad; jello for snack

    b. red beans and rice, fish sticks, pears; 1/2 cup Total cereal with milk for snack

    c. roast beef sandwich on rye bread, spinach salad, peach; raisins for snack

    d. chicken noodle soup, crackers, fruit cocktail; pudding cup for snack

59. Mr. Longjohn was recently diagnosed with leukemia and is receiving chemotherapy. His white cell count is low, so the RN is administering Neupogen® injections to boost his count. His daughter calls to schedule a visit and plans on bringing the granddaughter who she casually mentions has the sniffles. What advice should you give the daughter?

    a. Remind the daughter that due to his low white cell count, the client is prone to picking up infections more easily.

    b. Request that they visit another time when the granddaughter is not sick.

    c. Tell the daughter it is okay for her to visit as long as the granddaughter wears a mask.

    d. Tell the daughter to pick up some fresh fruit on the way to the home.

UNIT 18 RESPIRATORY SYSTEM

LEARNING OBJECTIVES

After studying this unit, you should be able to:

- Discuss the basic function of the respiratory system

- Name the major organs of the respiratory system

- Define and list common signs and symptoms of pneumonia, chronic bronchitis, asthma, and emphysema

- List two tests used to diagnose respiratory diseases

- Describe two devices used to administer oxygen

- Demonstrate the following:
  Procedure 71 Collecting a Sputum Specimen
  Procedure 72 Assisting with Cough and Deep-Breathing Exercises
  Procedure 73 Assisting the Client with Oxygen Therapy

TERMS TO DEFINE

- asthma
- chronic bronchitis
- chronic obstructive pulmonary disease (COPD)
- emphysema
- expectorate
- hypostatic
- nebulizer
- pneumonia
- pneumonia vaccine
- respiratory system

APPLICATION EXERCISES

Short Answer/Fill in the Blanks. *Complete the following sentences with the correct word or words.*

1. The respiratory system keeps the body supplied with _____.

2. Oxygen is carried by the blood to the cells of the body. At the same time, _____ _____ is picked up from the cells by the blood and taken to the lungs where it is removed from the body.

3. Breathing involves _____ which is inhaled, and _____ _____ which is exhaled.

4. The primary organs of the respiratory tract are the _____, pharynx, larynx, _____, bronchi, and _____.

5. Chronic obstructive pulmonary disease (_____) refers to the decreased ability of the lungs to perform the _____ function, which may result from an acute _____ such as pneumonia or a chronic condition such as bronchitis, _____, or emphysema.

6. Clients with breathing difficulties need more frequent _____ periods, more time to accomplish _____, and are often anxious.

7. Doctors often prescribe _____, bronchodilators, _____, or compressed or portable _____ containers for clients with breathing difficulties.

8. A _____ is a medical device power-driven by a compressed air machine that changes liquid medicine into a fine mist more effectively absorbed by the _____.

9. The home health aide assists in collecting a sputum specimen by encouraging the client to _____ _____, bring up mucus from the lungs, and _____ into a specimen container.

10. Pneumonia is an inflammation of the _____ due to an infection. It is a leading cause of _____ in the United States.

11. The _____ are particularly susceptible to pneumonia. The home health aide needs to be alert to the symptoms to inform the _____.

12. Symptoms of pneumonia include fever, _____ _____ with thick phlegm, sharp chest pain, _____ _____, nausea, vomiting, and fatigue.

13. The type of pneumonia seen in weak older adults and postsurgical clients is called _____ pneumonia due to inactivity of the lungs. Deep-breathing _____ and use of incentive spirometer device can prevent this type of pneumonia.

14. Preventive measures include yearly _____ shot and pneumonia _____.

15. Chronic bronchitis can result from asthma, bronchitis, _____ _____, and _____ _____.

16. Bronchitis is inflammation of the _____.

17. Four symptoms of bronchitis are:

   a. _____

   b. _____

   c. _____

   d. _____

18. Medications are given to the client with bronchitis to dilate the _____ and facilitate _____ _____.

19. A condition affecting the bronchial tubes or airways of the lungs caused by an allergic reaction is called _____.

20. Asthma is associated with _____ of large and small airways causing spasms.

21. Clients experiencing an asthma attack may have severe difficulty breathing, _____, sweating, feelings of suffocation, and _____.

22. The home health aide needs to help the client with respiratory distress to relax and remain _____.

23. The asthma treatment plan includes resolving immediate respiratory distress using a medication inhaler or _____ treatment, _____ of client torso, and encouraging the client to _____ through the nose and _____ through pursed lips.

24. A lung condition in which the air sacs within the lung lose their elasticity is called _____.

25. The typical emphysema client is a _____, 50 to 60 years of age.

26. Early symptoms of emphysema include shortness of breath, which gradually worsens, _____ breathing, and use of accessory muscles especially diaphragm; later symptoms include _____ chest, headache, _____, possible confusion due to poor _____ _____, and leaning forward in posture.

27. Part of the care plan for clients with emphysema is _____ as ordered to facilitate breathing. Too much oxygen for these clients can raise blood gas levels too high, therefore eliminating the _____ to breathe.

28. A position often used by the emphysema client is _____ _____ in a lounge chair, even sleeping in this position because it aids breathing.

29. The purpose of assisting the client with oxygen therapy is:

    a. _____

    b. _____

    c. _____

30. The client receiving oxygen therapy needs to have _____ mouth care.

31. The procedure for assisting clients with oxygen therapy includes checking that the client's oxygen gauge is set at prescribed _____ flow; checking to see if the client's oxygen mask or _____ is placed properly; checking tops of _____ and beneath _____ for signs of irritation; and checking that all _____ _____ are being observed.

32. List four safety precautions for clients using oxygen therapy.

    a. _____

    b. _____

    c. _____

    d. _____

True or False. *Answer the following statements true (T) or false (F).*

33. T   F   The respiratory system is made up of eyes, nose, mouth, esophagus, and lungs.
34. T   F   The respiratory system filters, warms, and humidifies the air we breathe.
35. T   F   People inhale carbon dioxide and exhale oxygen.
36. T   F   Emphysema is a leading cause of death in the United States.
37. T   F   A sputum specimen may be required to diagnose a respiratory illness.
38. T   F   Asthma involves swelling in the airways and increased mucus production.
39. T   F   Asthma control centers on reducing allergens.

Multiple Choice. *Choose the correct answer or answers.*

40. Clients with chronic respiratory difficulties will need
    a. a soft, comfortable chair   c. frequent rest periods
    b. a box of Kleenex   d. none of these

41. The role of the home health aide in breathing treatments includes
    a. preparing the medication
    b. instructing the client in the proper technique
    c. administering the breathing treatment
    d. observing the client for difficulties with the treatment

42. Pneumonia is dangerous to older adults because
    a. they have many chronic diseases   c. both a and b
    b. older adults are more vulnerable   d. none of these

43. Structures of the respiratory system include the
    a. heart and veins   c. kidneys, heart, and sinuses
    b. lungs, nose, and trachea   d. all of these

44. Assisting the client with deep-breathing exercises includes asking the client to
    a. take deep breaths through the nose   c. take a deep breath and cough
    b. hold the breath for 5 to 7 seconds   d. all of these

45. The home health aide's role in oxygen therapy includes
    a. instructing people not to smoke around oxygen c. applying lubricant to lips
    b. giving the client frequent mouth care   d. all of these

46. Collecting a sputum specimen involves
    a. washing hands and applying gloves; include mask if client has infectious disease
    b. obtaining specimen container; encourage client to breathe deeply then cough bringing up sputum from the lungs
    c. having client expectorate 1 to 2 tablespoons of sputum into container; apply lid and place in moisture-proof bag, and wash hands
    d. all of the above

47. Chronic bronchitis is

   a. an illness involving teenagers and young adults

   b. the result of an acute condition involving asthma, bronchitis, cigarette smoking, and air pollution

   c. inflammation of the bronchi

   d. inflammation of the aveoli

48. Pneumonia is

   a. an inflammation of the lungs due to an infection

   b. a lung condition in which the air sacs within the lung lose their elasticity

   c. diagnosed by chest x-rays and sputum analysis

   d. treated with antibiotics

49. Oxygen is delivered to clients

   a. through a concentrator that removes oxygen from room air

   b. through oxygen tanks delivered by an equipment company

   c. through a nebulizer machine

   d. all of the above

Documentation Exercises. *Read the following descriptions and provide documentation for each scenario.*

50. You are instructed to care for Mr. L. When you arrive to bathe him, you find him sitting in a chair. He is chain-smoking and has an oxygen cannula in his nose. You see a plastic tube that runs from his nose into the next room. In the next room, you locate his oxygen concentrator. You remind him that it is not safe to smoke around oxygen. He states it is safe because the oxygen is in the next room. What would you do? How would you document this information?

51. You are asked to obtain a sputum specimen from your client. Document this procedure.

Label the Diagram.

52. Label the parts of the respiratory system; refer to Figure 18–1.

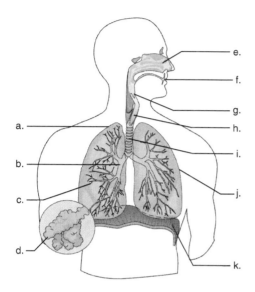

a. _____

b. _____

c. _____

d. _____

e. _____

f. _____

g. _____

h. _____

i. _____

j. _____

k. _____

Figure 18–1

PRACTICE SITUATIONS

Case 1

You arrive at Mrs. Katz's home. You find her sitting on the couch. She is gasping for breath. You check her vital signs. Her temperature is 101°F, her pulse is 100 and thready, and her respirations are 30.

Questions

1. What do you think is going on?
2. What do you need to do first?
3. Who would you contact?

Case 2

When you arrive at Mrs. Kasper's home, you find that her family is giving her a birthday party. In the front room, Mrs. Kasper is sitting on the couch with her oxygen cannula in place. Her son is sitting next to her smoking. They have brought a large cake and are serving it with ice cream. You know Mrs. Kasper is on a very strict diet. She looks at you and you can tell she does not know how to handle this situation.

Questions

1. What do you do first?
2. How will you handle the relatives without offending them?

CROSSWORD PUZZLE

Across

5 gas inhaled from the air

8 secretions expectorated from lungs

9 machine used to deliver fine mist medication to the lungs

10 condition affects bronchial tubes or airways of lung

12 device used to encourage deep breathing

Down

1 chronic inflammation of the bronchi

2 chronic obstructive pulmonary disease abbreviation

3 system made up of nose, pharynx, larynx, trachea, bronchi, and lungs

4 vaccine given to prevent pneumonia

6 lung condition in which air sacs within the lung lose elasticity

7 inflammation of the lungs due to an infection

11 spit up

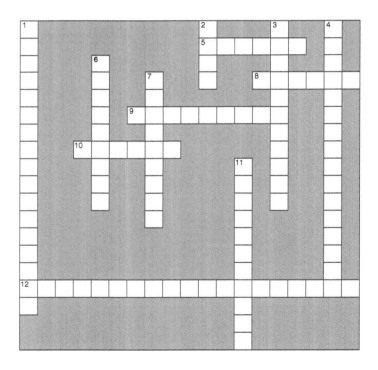

UNIT QUIZ

Fill in the Blanks. *Complete the following sentences with the correct word or words.*

1. Blood is supplied with fresh oxygen by means of _____ system.

2. Fresh air is _____ into the body and carried to the _____ then is carried to all parts of the body by the _____ system.

3. As oxygen is delivered to the cells of the body, waste gases mostly _____ _____ are picked up and carried back to the _____ and _____ from the body.

4. In addition to gas exchange, the respiratory system filters, warms, and humidifies the _____ we breathe.

5. Decreased ability of the lungs to perform the ventilation function affects those diseases called _____ _____ _____ _____.

6. Treatments prescribed for clients with lung disorders include _____, bronchodilators, nebulizers, compressors, or portable _____ containers.

7. Although the home health aide will not be teaching or administering a breathing treatment, it is important to observe and report to the health care team: _____ difficulties, difficulties using _____, or problems taking prescribed _____.

8. A leading cause of death in the United States is due to _____.

9. Treatment for pneumonia includes rest, _____, antibiotics, adequate _____, and possibly oxygen therapy.

10. Bronchitis is an inflammation of the _____.

11. A nebulizer changes liquid _____ into a fine mist that is absorbed more effectively by the lungs. The home health aide is not permitted to administer _____ treatments but can assist by gathering equipment.

12. It is recommended that older adults get a _____ shot because the flu can lead to pneumonia.

13. Sputum specimens should be from the _____ and not saliva from the _____.

14. Symptoms of _____ may include coughing, difficulty breathing, wheezing, and a feeling of tightness in the chest.

15. Clients should place expectorated mucus into _____, which are disposed of in a plastic bag as part of infection control measures.

True or False. *Answer the following statements true (T) or false (F).*

16. T   F   The respiratory system consists of the nose, pharynx, larynx, trachea, bronchi, and lungs.

17. T   F   Pneumonia is an acute infection of the lung.

18. T   F   Symptoms of chronic bronchitis include high-grade fever with productive cough, lethargy, and malaise.

19. T   F   The typical emphysema patient is a smoker.

20. T   F   The client should use mouthwash before collecting a sputum specimen.

Matching. *Match each term with the correct definition.*

21. _____ expectorate

22. _____ incentive spirometer

23. _____ nebulizer

24. _____ oxygen

25. _____ sputum

a. gas inhaled from the air

b. spit up

c. machine used to deliver fine mist medication to the lungs

d. secretions expectorated from lungs

e. device used to encourage deep breathing

Multiple Choice. *Choose the correct answer or answers.*

26. Inflammation of the lungs due to an infection is called

   a. pneumonia

   b. chronic bronchitis

   c. asthma

   d. emphysema

27. The home health aide needs to be aware of pneumonia symptoms in older adults because

   a. many older adults do not have severe early symptoms and can become acutely ill quickly

   b. many older adults already have preexisting conditions and chronic illness

   c. immune system of older adults is compromised

   d. all of the above

28. The type of pneumonia seen in weak older adults and postsurgical clients is called

   a. hypotension

   b. hypertension

   c. hypostatic

   d. hyperventilation

29. The home health aide assists with cough and deep-breathing exercises

   a. to prevent congestion or infections in the client's lungs

   b. to expand the lungs

   c. to give the client something to do while hospitalized

   d. to increase the barrel chest of client

30. When using an incentive spirometer

   a. inhale air through the mouthpiece of the device

   b. try to get the ball upwards as far as one can in the device, then hold for 6 to 7 seconds

   c. slowly exhale the air after removing the mouthpiece

   d. all of the above

31. The respiratory disorder that causes constriction of the bronchial tubes or airways of the lungs is called

   a. pneumonia

   b. chronic bronchitis

   c. asthma

   d. emphysema

32. List three things the home health aide can do to assist a client having an asthma attack.

   a.

   b.

   c.

33. Mr. McArthur fell and broke his leg. A home health aide is assigned to assist him with bathing. While assisting him, you note a barrel chest, shortness of breath, use of pursed-lip breathing, and use of accessory muscles to get into and out of the tub. You realize he has a preexisting illness called

   a. pneumonia   c. asthma

   b. chronic bronchitis   d. emphysema

34. The purpose of the home health aide in assisting the client with oxygen therapy includes

   a. to assist the client to receive the correct amount of oxygen

   b. to avoid misuse of oxygen equipment and careless practices that risk causing fires, explosions, or injury

   c. to aid in breathing

   d. to prevent oxygen from escaping the home

35. Safety precautions around oxygen include

   a. posting "No Smoking" sign at entrance to the home and warning visitors not to smoke in room where client is receiving oxygen

   b. not using matches, candles, or open flames where oxygen is used or stored

   c. avoiding sparks; do not use electrical appliances like electric shavers or woolen blankets, which may create static electricity

   d. all of the above

36. Clients with emphysema should use only the prescribed amount of oxygen as

   a. using too much oxygen is wasteful

   b. too much oxygen will raise carbon dioxide gas levels too high, eliminating the stimulus to breathe, resulting in death

   c. Medicare will not pay for excess oxygen used

   d. the client will run out of oxygen before next delivery

37. Because oxygen often dries out the mucous membranes of the nose and throat, it is often humidified. The humidifier should be filled when almost empty with

   a. chocolate milk   c. sterile water

   b. salt water   d. distilled water

38. Mrs. Kazanjian has COPD. The aide expects her care plan to include

   a. needing rest periods between activities because she tires easily

   b. needing more time to accomplish activities

   c. preparing lite foods to conserve energy stores

   d. for the aide to stay calm when client is having anxious episodes

39. Miss Hallahan has episodes several times a year of low-grade fever; coughing spells with thick white, greenish, or yellow phlegm; lethargy; malaise; and breathlessness. She has

   a. pneumonia   c. asthma

   b. chronic bronchitis   d. emphysema

40. The device used to concentrate oxygen from room air to administer to a client is called
    a. oxygen concentrator
    b. nebulizer
    c. portable oxygen tank
    d. incentive spirometer

41. When checking the oxygen device for prescribed setting the aide should check the dial for correct
    a. atmospheric pressure
    b. minutes of therapy
    c. volume
    d. liter flow

UNIT 19   REPRODUCTIVE SYSTEM

LEARNING OBJECTIVES

After studying this unit, you should be able to:
- Identify the male and female reproductive organs
- Describe the functions of each major organ
- List and describe male and female hormones and their functions
- Name three common disorders of the reproductive system
- List five sexually transmitted diseases and their symptoms
- Discuss how sexually transmitted diseases can be prevented

TERMS TO DEFINE

- cervix
- chlamydia
- dysmenorrhea
- ectopic pregnancy
- estrogen
- fallopian tubes
- genital herpes
- genital warts
- genitalia
- gonorrhea
- gynecologist
- menopause
- menstruation
- nongonococcal urethritis

- ovaries
- pelvic inflammatory disease (PID)
- penis
- progesterone
- scrotum
- sexually transmitted disease (STD)
- syphilis
- testes
- testosterone
- urethra
- uterus
- vagina
- vaginitis
- vulva

APPLICATION EXERCISES

Short Answer/Fill in the Blanks. *Complete the following sentences with the correct word or words.*

1. The male reproductive organs include the _____, the _____, the _____, and the hormone _____.

2. In the male, the _____ transports urine and sperm.

3. The female internal reproductive organs include the _____, the cervix, the _____, and the ovaries, which produce _____ and _____ hormones, and the fallopian tubes. The external organs are the genitalia and _____.

4. The mouth of the uterus is called the _____.

5. Menstruation is the sloughing off of the uterine _____. This occurs every _____ days if the egg is not fertilized.

6. The _____ that produce male and female characteristics are also thought to help maintain function in other systems of the body.

7. The pain females sometimes experience with menstruation is called _____. Treatment of pain is usually with nonsteroidal anti-inflammatory drugs (NSAIDs) for relief of discomfort.

8. Vaginitis can be caused by bacteria, viruses, or _____.

9. _____ usually has a white, odorous discharge with intense itching and burning.

10. Treatment for reproductive illnesses should by started only after the client has seen a _____.

11. Sexually transmitted diseases (STDs) are infections spread by _____ _____. Common symptoms occur in or near the vagina or penis and include: unusual _____; lumps, bumps, or rashes; _____ that are painful, itchy, or painless; itchy skin; _____ _____ _____.

12. In most cases _____ partners exposed to sexually transmitted diseases need to be tested and treated; if only one person is treated, that person can be _____ again if his or her partner is not treated.

13. _____ is a disease caused by bacteria that is spread when infected fluid from the sex organ or rectum contacts the penis, vagina, mouth, or anus.

14. Untreated bacterial infection may spread to the upper female reproductive tract, causing pelvic inflammatory disease and can result in _____; it can be treated with _____.

15. List four complications of pelvic inflammatory disease.

    a. _____

    b. _____

    c. _____

    d. _____

16. Gonorrhea, a bacterial infection, causes a discharge of _____ from the penis or sometimes the vagina, and pain on urination.

17. A pregnant female with gonorrhea risks passing the illness to the _____ during childbirth.

18. The earliest symptom of _____ is an ulcer on the genitals.

19. Syphilis progresses in three stages and becomes more _____ in each stage. Later effects of syphilis include brain, _____, and _____ disorders.

20. _____ _____ is a common STD and it tends to recur.

21. The first attack of herpes may be accompanied by _____, fever, and pain in the _____, _____, and _____.

22. People with herpes can relieve the symptoms with _____ _____ and _____.

23. People with the symptoms of an STD should _____ from sex. Their _____ should be checked for infection and also treated.

24. Genital warts are caused by _____. A wart may appear as a _____ or a small pink or red _____ that can be painful and irritating. Treatment includes chemicals, _____, or laser therapy; warts can continue to _____ and removing the warts _____ _____ mean the disease is cured.

25. List three ways to prevent sexually transmitted diseases.

   a. _____

   b. _____

   c. _____

True or False. *Answer the following statements true (T) or false (F).*

26. T   F   Sexually transmitted diseases are spread by casual contact.

27. T   F   Vaginitis is an infection of the cervix.

28. T   F   Pelvic inflammatory disease is generally a result of an STD.

29. T   F   Antiviral medications are a cure for herpes.

30. T   F   Sexually active people should practice safe sex.

Multiple Choice. *Choose the correct answer or answers.*

31. Pelvic inflammatory disease can be caused by

   a. pneumonia   c.   chlamydia

   b. gonorrhea   d.   both b and c

32. Small blisters on the penis and around the vagina are symptoms of

   a. herpes   c.   AIDS

   b. gonorrhea   d.   none of these

33. There is no cure for

   a. AIDS   c.   syphilis

   b. gonorrhea   d.   pneumonia

34. Pain that sometimes accompanies menstrual flow is called

   a. vaginitis   c.   dysmenorrhea

   b. gonorrhea   d.   nausea

35. A sac-like male organ that contains the testes is called the

   a. cervix   c.   urethra

   b. rectum   d.   scrotum

36. The testes produce
    a. sperm
    b. testosterone
    c. fluid
    d. all of the above

37. The male urethra transports
    a. urine
    b. egg cells
    c. sperm
    d. saliva

38. The uterus is located behind the urinary bladder and functions as
    a. the womb that receives the fertilized egg
    b. the tube that carries egg cells
    c. the birth canal
    d. all of the above

39. The hormone that produces male characteristics such as broad shoulders, facial, chest, and pubic hair is
    a. testosterone
    b. testis
    c. estrogen
    d. progesterone

40. The ovaries produce which substances?
    a. estrogen
    b. progesterone
    c. egg cells
    d. all of the above

Documentation Exercises. *Read the following descriptions and provide documentation for each scenario.*

41. You are assigned to care for Mr. Jon, who has recently had a catheter placed into his bladder. While you are bathing him, you notice urine on the bed sheet. Checking the catheter, you see pus-like drainage from the head of the penis. What do you need to do? How do you document this finding?

42. Your client, Mr. Tote, has a diagnosis of genital herpes. You are required to give Mr. Tote a bed bath; he is unable to assist you. You know that you need to wear gloves and follow good universal precautions. How do you document this care?

Label the Diagram.

43. Label the parts of the male reproductive system on the diagram; refer to Figure 19–1.

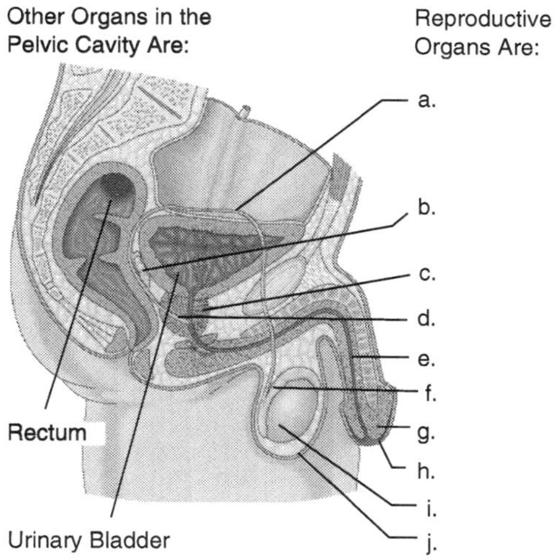

Other Organs in the Pelvic Cavity Are:
Reproductive Organs Are:
a.
b.
c.
d.
e.
f.
g.
h.
i.
j.
Rectum
Urinary Bladder
Figure 19–1

a. ______
b. ______
c. ______
d. ______
e. ______
f. ______
g. ______
h. ______
i. ______
j. ______

44. Label the parts of the female reproductive system on the diagram; refer to Figure 19–2.

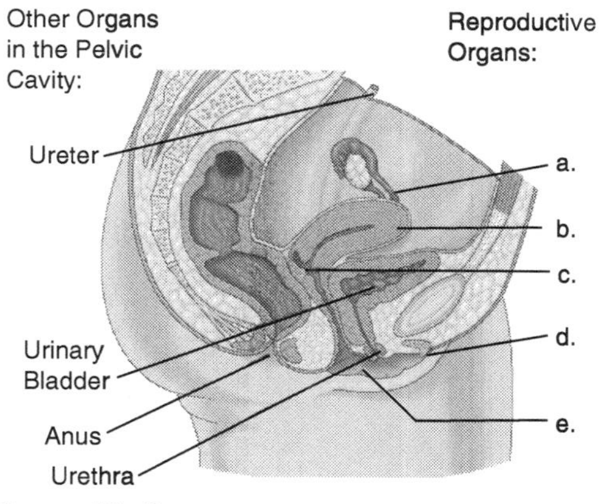

Other Organs in the Pelvic Cavity:
Reproductive Organs:
Ureter
a.
b.
c.
d.
e.
Urinary Bladder
Anus
Urethra
Figure 19–2

a. ______
b. ______
c. ______
d. ______
e. ______

45. Label the parts of the female reproductive system on the diagram; refer to Figure 19–3.

a.
b.
c.
d.
e.
f.
g.
Figure 19–3

a. ______
b. ______
c. ______
d. ______
e. ______
f. ______
g. ______

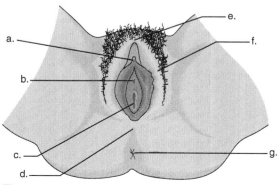

PRACTICE SITUATIONS

Case 1

You have been caring for Mrs. Phillips for several months. When you change her bed, you notice blood on the sheets. You ask her where the bleeding is coming from. She tells you that after all these years, she is having a period again. You know something is wrong because Mrs. Phillips is 85 years old.

Questions

1. What would you tell her about the bleeding?

2. Who would you call?

3. What do you think is wrong?

Case 2

Mr. Tomas has recently had a prostatectomy. You know that this surgery affects his ability to have sexual relations. He asks you when he will be able to have sex with his wife again.

Questions

1. How will you answer him?

2. What can you tell him?

3. Who else do you need to inform about this situation?

CROSSWORD PUZZLE

Across

2 permanent end of menstruation

5 vulva

6 sac-like organ that contains testes

9 birth canal

11 bacterial infection causing discharge of pus

13 organ that produces sperm

15 pain experienced during menstruation

17 infection of upper female reproductive tract

Down

1 contains the male urethra

3 release egg cells and female hormones

4 infections spread by sexual intercourse

7 womb

8 carry egg cells from ovaries to uterus

10 male hormone

12 female hormone

14 egg cell grows in fallopian tube

16 infection starts with ulcer on genitals

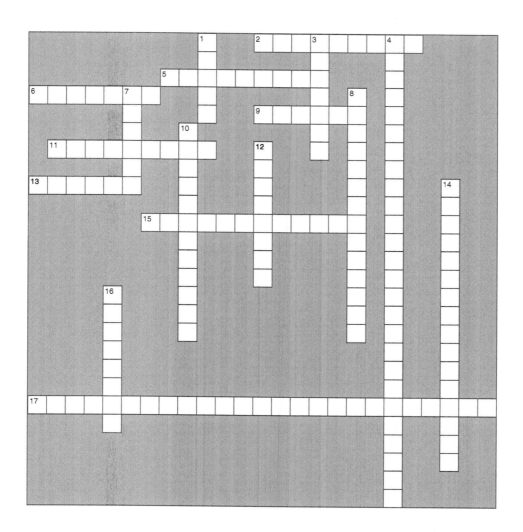

UNIT QUIZ

Fill in the Blanks. *Complete the following sentences with the correct word or words.*

1. The internal and external sex organs of the male and female make up the
_____ system.

2. The external female reproductive organs are the _____ and
_____.

3. The external male reproductive organs are the _____ and
_____ while the internal organs are the _____ and
_____.

4. Illness or malfunction of the reproductive system can cause _____ and
_____ problems.

5. The female reproductive cycle is about 28 days long in which the uterus prepares for a
fertilized egg. If the egg cell is not fertilized, the uterine lining sloughs off with bleeding
occurring for three to five days. This process is called _____.

6. Common disorders of the female reproductive system include _____,
vaginitis, and changes in _____ secretions after menopause.

7. A prevalent STD, _____ _____ results in urethral
inflammation caused by an infection other than gonorrhea.

8. One of the most common STDs is _____ _____ caused by the
herpes simplex virus. Crops of small blisters form on the penis or around the
_____ then develop into shallow _____.

9. Herpes symptoms include small _____ formation on the penis or vagina with
the first attack accompanied by headache, _____, and pain in the groin,
buttocks and legs.

10. Treatment of genital herpes focuses on pain relief and _____ drugs.

11. The main sites of gonorrhea infection include the _____ in males and the
_____ in females with main symptom discharge of _____.

12. Pain experienced during menstruation is called _____ and is most often
relieved with nonsteroidal anti-inflammatory drugs (NSAIDs).

13. In females, the urethral orifice is located _____ the vaginal orifice.

14. In men, gonorrhea infects the _____ and then spreads to the
_____ and prostrate causing pain, swelling, and scarring.

True or False. *Answer the following statements true (T) or false (F).*

15. T F Dysmenorrhea refers to pain that sometimes accompanies the menstrual flow.

16. T F One of the most common sexually transmitted diseases, genital herpes is easily cured.

17. T F STDs have become more prevalent in recent years.

18. T F Syphilis, if left untreated, will advance to the later stage affecting the brain.

Matching. *Match each term with the correct definition.*

19. ____ scrotum

20. ____ vagina

21. ____ testosterone

22. ____ urethra

23. ____ fallopian tubes

24. ____ cervix

25. ____ menstruation

26. ____ estrogen

27. ____ ovaries

28. ____ testes

29. ____ penis

a. saclike organ contains testes

b. birth canal

c. male hormone

d. organ that carries urine and sperm

e. carry egg cells from ovaries to uterus

f. mouth of the uterus

g. process of monthly uterine lining sloughing

h. female hormone

i. release egg cells and hormones

j. produce sperm

k. contains the male urethra

Multiple Choice. *Choose the correct answer or answers.*

30. The male reproductive organs include all of the following except

    a. scrotum

    b. testes

    c. testosterone

    d. breasts

31. The female reproductive internal organs include all of the following except

    a. vagina

    b. cervix

    c. uterus

    d. breasts

32. Testosterone hormone produces the male characteristics of

    a. broad shoulders

    b. height

    c. facial, chest, and pubic hair

    d. all of the above

33. The hormones responsible for female characteristics such as rounded hips, enlarged breasts, and pubic hair are

    a. insulin

    b. estrogen

    c. testosterone

    d. sperm

34. A health care provider specializing in women's reproductive health is called a

    a. cardiologist

    b. beautician

    c. proctologist

    d. gynecologist

35. Prevention of sexually transmitted diseases focuses on

    a. having a single sex partner

    b. always using a condom when engaged in penetrative sex

    c. frequent douching

    d. bathing after sexual intercourse

36. A bacterial infection causing a discharge of pus from the penis or vagina plus pain on urination is called

    a. gonorrhea

    b. pelvic inflammatory disease

    c. genital herpes

    d. syphilis

37. Many sexually transmitted diseases can be treated with

    a. heat therapy

    b. antibiotics

    c. analgesics

    d. anti-inflammatory drugs

38. Vaginitis treatment consists of all of the following except

    a. wearing cotton underwear and avoiding garments that hold heat and moisture

    b. eating yogurt

    c. treating infectious organisms with drugs

    d. douching

39. You are assisting bathing Mrs. Adamson who broke both legs in a car accident 10 days ago. She is wearing a hip spica cast. You notice an odorous, thick white, cheesecake-like drainage from the client's vagina, and Mrs. Adamson says it burns and itches. You report the symptoms to the nurse and suspect she has

    a. vaginitis

    b. gonorrhea

    c. syphilis

    d. genital herpes

40. Mr. Clement was known as quite a "ladies man" when he was younger. He is admitted to home care after having a mild CVA. Four weeks later, he remains very forgetful and has difficulty with coordination. You are hired to assist with personal care. His health care provider is concerned that his forgetfulness hasn't resolved and orders some blood tests. The test for sexually transmitted diseases is positive, all others are normal. Mr. Clement has signs of advanced

    a. vaginitis

    b. gonorrhea

    c. syphilis

    d. genital herpes

41. Mr. Truman has advanced multiple sclerosis, and is catheterized. While performing catheter care, you observe a small crop of blisters on the penis. He tells you he is having an outbreak of

    a. vaginitis

    b. gonorrhea

    c. syphilis

    d. genital herpes

42. You have been hired to care for Ms. Lovett who is pregnant and on bed rest due to uterine bleeding. She confides in you she has had difficulty conceiving and miscarried in the past due to pelvic inflammatory disease (PID) when she was in her late teens. One day she complains of severe right-sided pain that doesn't go away with repositioning or pain medication. You call 911 at her request and are concerned that she might be having the following complication of PID

    a. ectopic pregnancy

    b. gonorrhea

    c. syphilis

    d. genital warts

43. Miss Partridge needs assistance with bathing due to Parkinson's disease. While performing perineal care, you notice several small pink and red growths along her labia. She tells you they have been removed in the past but recently reappeared. You realize she has

    a. ectopic pregnancy

    b. gonorrhea

    c. syphilis

    d. genital warts

44. While caring for a client with a sexually transmitted disease, the home health aide should do all but

    a. Assist the client with pelvic exercises.

    b. Wash hands before and after providing care.

    c. Wear gloves.

    d. Change the bathwater after bathing genitalia.

UNIT 20   ENDOCRINE SYSTEM AND DIABETES

LEARNING OBJECTIVES

After studying this unit, you should be able to:

- List six glands of the endocrine system
- Discuss the importance of hormones
- List two disorders of the thyroid gland
- Name four signs and symptoms of diabetes
- List four types of diabetes mellitus
- Name three ways of controlling diabetes
- Name three long-term complications of diabetes
- List signs and symptoms for hypoglycemia and hyperglycemia and the immediate care for each
- Explain special foot care given to the diabetic client
- Describe special techniques used in caring for a client who has vision impairment
- Demonstrate the following:
  Procedure 73   Testing Blood

TERMS TO DEFINE

- acidosis
- blood lancet
- cyanotic
- diabetes
- diabetic coma
- ducts
- endocrine glands
- gangrene
- gestational
- glucometer
- glucose
- hormone
- hyperglycemia
- hyperthyroidism
- hypoglycemia
- hypothyroidism
- insulin
- insulin shock
- neuropathy
- subcutaneously

APPLICATION EXERCISES

Short Answer/Fill in the Blanks. *Complete the following sentences with the correct word or words.*

1. The _____ _____ is composed of many _____ scattered throughout the body.

2. Chemicals that are secreted by the endocrine glands directly into the bloodstream are called _____.

3. These secretions are carried by the blood or lymph system to all parts of the body to _____ and _____ body functions.

4. The _____ _____ regulates the metabolic rate of the body.

5. People with hyperthyroidism have a _____ heartbeat and tend to be _____ and irritable.

6. Clients with an underactive thyroid tend to be sluggish and _____ _____ easily. This disorder can be easily treated with thyroid drugs.

7. Diabetes mellitus is a _____ disease with no _____; it is primarily managed through _____, exercise, and _____ therapy.

8. The functions of insulin are to enable the body to use _____ (sugar), to aid in the storage of nutrients, and to make possible the metabolism of _____ and protein.

9. Diabetes develops when _____ is not produced by the body. The _____ either does not produce any or produces an inadequate amount of insulin.

10. List five risk factors for developing diabetes.

   a. _____

   b. _____

   c. _____

   d. _____

   e. _____

11. _____ is the third leading cause of death by disease in the United States.

12. The three main types of diabetes are:

   a. _____

   b. _____

   c. _____

13. Insulin-dependent diabetes mellitus (type I) usually occurs in people before age 25 when the pancreas no longer produces any _____. Clients need to take _____ _____ _____ to stay alive.

14. _____ – _____ – _____ diabetes (type II) usually develops after the age of 40 and is common in the older adults. Insulin is produced but in _____ amounts. People usually take _____ medication but may need insulin.

15. Gestational diabetes occurs during a woman's _____ and usually returns to normal after delivery. These women often will develop diabetes later in life unless changes are made in _____ and _____.

16. Five signs and symptoms of diabetes are:

    a. _____

    b. _____

    c. _____

    d. _____

    e. _____

17. Blood testing using a _____ is the best method to control diabetes.

18. The home health aide needs to be alert to signs of _____ and _____ and always report these signs to the nurse.

19. Normal blood sugar is between _____ mg to _____ mg.

20. If a blood sugar goes too low, a condition called _____ occurs, also known as _____ _____. This condition occurs due to an imbalance between _____ _____ and dosage of insulin or oral medications.

21. List five signs of hypoglycemia.

    a. _____

    b. _____

    c. _____

    d. _____

    e. _____

22. A blood sugar under _____ is considered an emergency. If the client is alert, the home health aide should give the client some form of _____ _____ such as hard candy, juice, honey, or glucose tablets.

23. A high blood sugar over 250 mg is called _____, also called diabetic _____ or coma. This condition occurs because of _____, too little insulin medication, emotional stress, or lack of _____.

24. Five signs of hyperglycemia are:

    a. _____

    b. _____

    c. _____

    d. _____

    e. _____

25. Untreated hyperglycemia may lead to the client becoming unresponsive; if this occurs, the home health aide should call _____.

26. If either insulin reaction or acidosis is not corrected immediately, _____ or _____ can occur.

27. _____ is the cornerstone to the management of diabetes.

28. Food intake for the diabetic should be distributed _____
_____ _____ and accommodate the client's lifestyle,
_____, and diabetic medication.

29. The _____ _____ _____ has developed
exchange lists of foods that can assist the aide and the client in meal planning.

30. An important duty of the home health aide is to _____ _____
using the diet prepared by the dietician along with reinforcing the importance of sticking to
this diet with the client.

31. Two common problems in diabetes are _____ and _____
_____.

32. Exercise can improve the client's _____, assist in maintaining
_____, increase the client's sense of _____, and improve
control of _____ in the body.

33. The home health aide plays an important role with the diabetic client by
_____ him or her to comply with requirements for exercise, especially if the
client is discouraged.

34. Type I diabetes is always treated with a drug called _____, which needs to be
injected _____ (under the skin).

35. Insulin cannot be taken orally because the stomach juices will _____ it.

36. A home health aide is _____ permitted to inject insulin.

37. The home health aide can help the client by bringing the bottle of _____ and
needed supplies to the client.

38. A new device for injecting insulin over time is called the insulin _____.

39. Name the three ways type II diabetes can be treated.

    a. _____

    b. _____

    c. _____

40. Oral hypoglycemic medications work in different ways to assist the client to
_____ _____ _____.

41. As a home health aide, it is important to encourage the client to take the medicine as it is
_____.

42. Abnormal conditions that occur after a client develops diabetes are called
_____ _____.

43. The most common complications are _____ (blood vessel) disease and a high
risk of _____.

44. Neuropathy is defined as a destructive disorder of the _____.

45. Diabetic neuropathy is the loss of sensation in the _____ with the client
unable to feel _____ or distinguish between hot and cold
_____.

46. It is important for the home health aide to check the client's lower extremities and
_____ every time the aide provides care for signs of redness, any
_____ area, swelling, or cracked or open skin cuts.

47. Trimming the toenails of a diabetic client must be performed by a _____.

48. Any abnormality of the feet or legs should be reported to the _____.

49. The diabetic client's feet should be cleansed with a mild _____, _____ with a soft towel, then a lanolin-based _____ applied.

50. List five foot care guidelines to reduce foot injury in the diabetic client.

    a. _____

    b. _____

    c. _____

    d. _____

    e. _____

51. The risk of infection in the diabetic client is increased because the high _____ in the blood helps bacteria to grow.

52. Hot and reddened areas of the skin are the first sign of _____.

53. A large area of dead skin tissue is called _____.

54. Loss of vision is a common problem of _____ _____ _____.

True or False. *Answer the following statements true (T) or false (F).*

55. T   F   Hormones are powerful substances.

56. T   F   Adrenalin causes the heart to slow down.

57. T   F   Diabetes is the third leading cause of death in the United States.

58. T   F   More than 11 million people in the United States have diabetes and almost half of them do not know it.

59. T   F   Insulin-dependent diabetes usually occurs after the age of 25.

60. T   F   Pregnant women always develop diabetes.

61. T   F   Exercise, alcohol, or decreased kidney functions can make hypoglycemia worse.

62. T   F   Improperly treated diabetes can lead to complications.

63. T   F   Walking barefoot in the house is okay for diabetic clients, as long as they are careful.

64. T   F   A diabetic client who develops acidosis, or insulin shock, needs to be informed to call his health care provider for an appointment.

Multiple Choice. *Choose the correct answer or answers.*

65. The gland called the master gland is the

    a. thyroid   c. pituitary

    b. adrenal   d. thymus

66. The metabolic rate of the body is regulated by which gland?

    a. thyroid   c. pituitary

    b. adrenal   d. thymus

67. The function of insulin is to help the body

    a. fight infection   c. grow in height

    b. use sugar   d. none of these

68. The type of diabetes that occurs during pregnancy in some women is called
    a. gestational
    b. insulin-dependent
    c. non–insulin-dependent
    d. all of these

69. Signs and symptoms that may indicate diabetes include
    a. frequent urination
    b. excessive thirst
    c. sores that do not heal
    d. all of these

70. Foods that the diabetic client should avoid or eat in small amounts include
    a. green leafy vegetables
    b. citrus fruit juices
    c. cakes and candies
    d. both b and c

71. Diabetics need to avoid foods with concentrated sugar. Clients should avoid all of the following except
    a. pies, cakes, and cookies
    b. canned fruit in heavy syrup
    c. breads, grains, and cereals
    d. regular jams and jellies

72. Rapid metabolism of food, rapid heartbeat, restlessness, and irritability are signs of
    a. hypothyroidism
    b. hyperthyroidism
    c. aldosteronism
    d. hyperparathyroidism

73. This hormone regulates sleep and wakefulness
    a. melatonin
    b. insulin
    c. synthroid
    d. estrogen

74. Home health aides provide the following diabetic foot care techniques except for
    a. Bathe the feet daily in warm, not hot water, then pat the feet dry with a soft towel, especially between the toes.
    b. Massage lotion into the feet starting at the toes and working toward the ankles to moisturize skin and increase circulation.
    c. Apply clean, white cotton socks and change daily.
    d. Cut toenails straight across to prevent ingrown toenails.

Documentation Exercises. *Read the following descriptions and provide documentation for each scenario.*

75. Mrs. Macy, your client, has diabetes and recently had to have an amputation of her lower left leg. When you arrive, you find her in the kitchen. She is eating sweet rolls. You greet her and ask her if the sweet roll is dietetic. She tells you that she is allowed to eat sweet rolls as long as she does not put sugar on them. What would you do? Document this discussion.

76. Mrs. Tam is an insulin-dependent diabetic. She has been diabetic for a short time. You are caring for her because she recently fractured her leg and needs help bathing. She informs you that she has been vomiting all night and is concerned that you will have to clean up the mess. She says, "I took my insulin just like I was supposed to." What do you say to her? Do you need to report this information to your case manager? Document this.

Label the Diagram.

77. Label the endocrine glands in the diagram; refer to Figure 20–1.

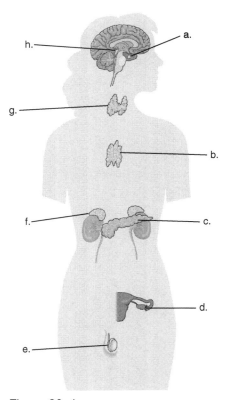

a. _____

b. _____

c. _____

d. _____

e. _____

f. _____

g. _____

h. _____

Figure 20–1

78. Label the parts of the endrocrine system in the diagram; Figure 20–2.

a. _____

b. _____

c. _____

d. _____

e. _____

f. _____

g. _____

h. _____

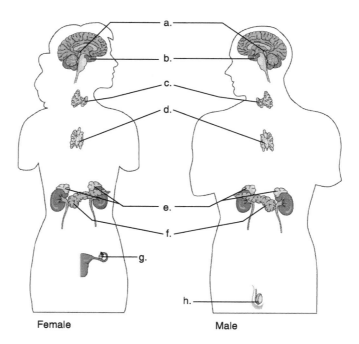

Female   Male

Figure 20–2

PRACTICE SITUATIONS

Case 1

You are caring for a new client, Mrs. Luau. She is diabetic and takes insulin every day. When you arrive, you ask her if she has taken her insulin. She informs you that she is out of insulin. She then asks you to purchase it for her. You tell her that you cannot purchase her insulin. She tells you that the other home health aides and nurses buy it for her. You know that she can afford to buy the insulin.

Questions

1. What do you do?

2. How will she get her insulin?

3. Who will you call?

Case 2

Mr. Lei is your new client. You have been assigned to bathe him and assist him in dressing. He takes a shower. When you are assisting him with his clothing, you notice that he has two rather large blisters on his left foot. When you ask him about them, he tells you not to worry about them because he gets them all the time. You know that he is diabetic and that wounds tend to be difficult to heal on diabetics.

Questions

1. What do you do?

2. Do you need to do any special treatment to the blisters?

3. Is there anything you can do to prevent further injury to the blisters?

CROSSWORD PUZZLE

Across

3 blood sugar less than 60 mg

6 blood testing equipment

8 elevated blood sugar above 250 mg

11 non–insulin-dependent diabetes mellitus

13 blue skin color

14 overactive thyroid

15 injected under the skin

Down

1 large area of dead tissue

2 hormone that helps the body use glucose

3 underactive thyroid

4 insulin-dependent diabetes mellitus

5 destructive disorder of the nerves

7 chemical secreted into the bloodstream

9 ductless glands that secrete hormones

10 diabetic coma

12 chronic disease due to lack of insulin

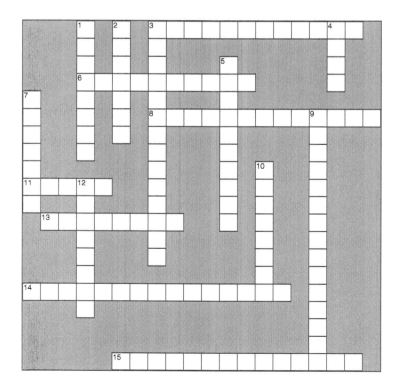

UNIT QUIZ

Short Answer/Fill in the Blanks. *Complete the following sentences with the correct word or words.*

1. Ductless glands that secrete hormones within the body are called _____ _____.

2. Hormones are _____ that are secreted directly into the _____.

3. The purpose of hormones is to _____ and _____ specific body functions.

4. People with sluggishness, fatigue, and chronically cold hands or feet may have a condition called _____ and can be treated with thyroid medication.

5. Hyperthyroidism is due to an _____ _____ _____ with persons experiencing rapid heartbeat, restlessness, and irritability.

6. _____ _____ develops when insulin is not manufactured or cannot be used correctly.

7. Functions of insulin include enabling the body to use _____, aiding in the storage of nutrients, and making possible the metabolism of _____ and protein.

8. The three main types of diabetes are:

    a. _____

    b. _____

    c. _____

9. List five signs of hypoglycemia.

    a. _____

    b. _____

    c. _____

    d. _____

    e. _____

10. List five signs of hyperglycemia.

    a. _____

    b. _____

    c. _____

    d. _____

    e. _____

True or False. *Answer the following statements true (T) or false (F).*

11. T   F   Diet is an important part of managing diabetes.

12. T   F   Hypoglycemia occurs when the blood sugar goes too high.

13. T   F   Men over the age of 40 are most often affected by hypothyroidism.

14. T   F   Adrenalin causes the heart rate to increase and speed up the body's reflexes.

15. T   F   Approximately 5 million Americans do not know they have diabetes.

16. T F Insulin shock occurs when the blood sugar is less than 50 mg, which requires emergency treatment.

17. T F Type I diabetes is never treated with insulin, only oral hypoglycemic medication.

18. T F A blood lancet is used by the client to obtain blood from fingers or arm for glucometer testing.

19. T F Insulin is injected subcutaneously into the muscles.

Matching. *Match each definition with the correct term.*

20. ____ secretes hormones that regulate many bodily processes

21. ____ regulates metabolic rate and growth process

22. ____ regulates metabolism of calcium and phosphorus

23. ____ adjust body to crisis and stress

24. ____ secrete estrogen and progesterone

25. ____ secrete testosterone

26. ____ produces insulin

27. ____ regulates immunity to infectious disease during infancy

28. ____ regulates secretion of melatonin

29. ____ hormone that helps the body to use glucose

a. adrenal

b. insulin

c. ovaries

d. pancreas

e. parathyroid

f. pineal

g. pituitary

h. testes

i. thymus

j. thyroid

Multiple Choice. *Choose the correct answer or answers.*

30. A symptom of diabetes is
    a. unusual thirst
    b. frequent need to urinate
    c. weakness
    d. all of these

31. The device used to measure a client's blood sugar level is called
    a. incentive spirometer
    b. thermometer
    c. glucometer
    d. pedometer

32. Hormones
    a. are chemicals secreted directly into the bloodstream
    b. are chemicals secreted through ducts (little tubes) into body organs
    c. regulate and control specific body functions
    d. in small amounts can trigger a body reaction

33. You have been caring for wheelchair-bound Mrs. Tang for six months. She confides in you that her 12-year-old daughter has been very cranky, frequently in the kitchen drinking water, gets up during the night to use the bathroom, and has lost weight. You have observed her daughter scratching her arms. Mrs. Tang asks you, "What could be the problem with my daughter?" You realize these are signs of

   a. hypothyroidism

   b. hyperthyroidism

   c. gestational diabetes

   d. diabetes mellitus

34. What should you do next about Mrs. Tang's concerns?

   a. Recommend that her daughter obtain a glucometer machine from the pharmacy to test her blood.

   b. Tell Mrs. Tang that her daughter should be seen by a health care provider immediately.

   c. Call 911.

   d. Notify the nurse about the client's concerns.

35. Mr. Jones receives home health aide assistance due to diabetic retinopathy and arthritis. Arriving at his home at 10 A.M., the home health aide finds the client shaking and unable to answer questions as to how he's feeling. Touching his arm to get his attention, the aide finds cold, clammy skin, rapid and weak pulse, and realizes the client is having signs of

   a. hypoglycemia

   b. hyperglycemia

   c. hypothyroidism

   d. hyperthyroidism

36. What should the aide do first regarding Mr. Jones's symptoms?

   a. Gather the glucometer equipment to test the client's blood sugar.

   b. Give the client some form of concentrated sugar such as juice, hard candy, honey, or glucose tablets.

   c. Call 911.

   d. Notify the nurse.

37. Mr. Hightower has been observed by the home health aide injecting insulin in the same site during the past five visits. What advice can the aide offer the client?

   a. Sites recommended for injection include the abdomen, upper arms, and thighs.

   b. Clients are encouraged to rotate injection sites on a daily or weekly basis to avoid changes in the skin tissues, which can alter the rate of absorption of the drug.

   c. Keeping a record of where the injection was given assists the client in rotating sites.

   d. All of the above.

38. Miss Mitchell has diabetic neuropathy. What must the home health aide be concerned about?

   a. client may be unable to feel pain or tell the difference between hot or cold temperatures

   b. cuts or wounds are not felt and thus not cared for; they can become easily infected

   c. many diabetics have poor eyesight or have difficulty bending and rely on the home health aide to check their feet

   d. all of the above

39. Home health aides carefully and routinely must check the diabetic client's feet and legs for

    a. any sign of redness or "warm" area

    b. any blueness or swelling of the ankles

    c. dry, scaly, itching, or cracked skin or any open cuts

    d. all of the above

40. The home health aide can reinforce diabetic foot care instructions, which include all except

    a. Bathe the feet daily in warm, not hot water, then pat the feet dry with a soft towel, especially between the toes.

    b. Massage lotion into the feet, starting at the toes and working toward the ankles to moisturize skin and increase circulation.

    c. Wear clean, white cotton socks and change daily.

    d. Seek treatment by a podiatrist for bunions and corns.

    e. Walking barefoot is permitted only in the home.

41. Coming back to care for Mr. Hilltop after a two-week vacation, you notice that his right foot, which was reddened, is now cold and bluish. He has a very dark and hard heel area. You suspect Mr. Hilltop has developed

    a. diabetic neuropathy

    b. diabetic acidosis

    c. gangrene

    d. diabetic retinopathy

42. After your observations of Mr. Hilltop's foot, you need to

    a. Call 911.

    b. Document your findings in your notes.

    c. Report your findings to the client's nurse.

    d. Tell the client to call his health care provider.

43. Mrs. Garcia has been feeling poorly for a few days since getting a cold. She has limited her activities due to weakness, abdominal cramps, slight nausea and vomiting, and generalized aches and pains. Upon your arrival to the home, you notice a fruity odor to her breath. You gather her glucometer supplies. Mrs. Garcia checks her blood sugar, with the reading 475 mg. Her symptoms indicate

    a. diabetic neuropathy

    b. diabetic acidosis

    c. gangrene

    d. diabetic retinopathy

44. What do you understand about Mrs. Garcia's blood sugar level?

    a. Call your supervisor immediately to report your findings, as it is a medical emergency.

    b. Insulin is needed as well as fluid replacements and blood tests to evaluate the client's metabolism.

    c. If acidosis is not corrected immediately, coma or death can occur.

    d. All of the above.

45. The home health aide understands that diabetics have problems with small cuts or abrasions healing because

    a. slow healing is due in part to poor circulation

    b. breakdown of the blood vessels prevents nutrients from being carried to the injured tissues and this delays healing

    c. risk of infection increases because of extra sugar in the blood, which promotes bacteria multiplying quickly

    d. all of the above

46. All diabetics should wear a Medic Alert identification tag, which includes all except

    a. name, address, and phone number   c. health care provider's name

    b. medical condition   d. blood type

47. Miss Ngyen never seems to gain weight. Recently, she has been restless, irritable, and feels like her heart is racing. The aide checks her pulse, which is rapid. She has signs and symptoms of

    a. hypoglycemia   c. hypothyroidism

    b. hyperglycemia   d. hyperthyroidism

48. Mrs. Smithfield tells the aide she just can't get moving anymore because she's tired and sluggish. She asks you to turn up the heat due to cold feet and hands. Recently, you've observed her puffy face, hoarse voice, and slight weight gain. These are symptoms of

    a. hypoglycemia   c. hypothyroidism

    b. hyperglycemia   d. hyperthyroidism

SECTION 6

Clients Requiring Special Care

UNIT 21   CARING FOR THE CLIENT WHO IS TERMINALLY ILL

LEARNING OBJECTIVES

After studying this unit, you should be able to:

- Explain the hospice program
- Discuss advanced directives
- Describe the five stages of grief
- Discuss the home health aide's responsibilities in providing supportive care and keeping the client pain-free
- List the physical signs of approaching death
- Identify ways in which a person may react to the death of a family member or friend
- Briefly describe major religious beliefs related to death and dying
- Explain the importance of grieving

TERMS TO DEFINE

- advance directives
- autopsy
- comatose
- durable power of attorney
- embalming
- grieving
- hospice
- living will
- mottling
- palliative
- Patient Self-Determination Act
- terminal

APPLICATION EXERCISES

Short Answer/Fill in the Blanks. *Complete the following sentences with the correct word or words.*

1. Most people in our society are uncomfortable talking or thinking about _____.

2. Families are now allowing their loved ones to die at _____ instead of a hospital.

3. _____ _____ is a choice for individuals who have been given a diagnosis that death will most likely come within the next six months.

4. Name the members of the hospice team.

   a. _____

   b. _____

   c. _____

   d. _____

   e. _____

5. The goal of _____ is to assist the client and family to make the dying process as pain-free and comfortable as possible.

6. The hospice team also helps the client with _____, financial, and _____ concerns.

7. _____ _____ emphasizes quality of life, not prolonging life.

8. The Patient Self-Determination Act is a law passed to allow clients to make a decision about the use of _____ _____.

9. _____ _____ are written directions that specify the type of treatment clients want or do not want under serious medical conditions in which they may be unable to communicate their wishes to the health care provider or family.

10. Advanced directives can be done by a living _____ or by a durable power of _____.

11. To enter a hospice program, a health care provider needs to certify that the client's _____ is less than six months due to a _____ _____.

12. The home health aide needs to respect the family's _____ in dealing with the death of a loved one.

13. Five stages of grief described by Dr. Elisabeth Kübler-Ross include:

    a. _____

    b. _____

    c. _____

    d. _____

    e. _____

14. The last sense to be lost is _____, so be careful what is said in the unconscious client's presence.

15. When the client knows there is no cure for his or her illness, the care given to the client is called _____ _____.

16. Palliative care emphasizes _____ _____ _____, not prolonging life.

17. Three home health aide responsibilities in caring for the dying client are:

    a. _____

    b. _____

    c. _____

18. There are many _____ available to keep the client as pain-free as possible.

19. Pain management is a cornerstone of hospice care. When a client is first started on pain medication, _____ _____ usually work better and are easier to take and less costly. As the disease progresses and the pain increases, _____ drugs are given.

20. It is best to keep _____ _____ _____ pain and take pain medication on a regular basis.

21. If clients are unable to take pain medication by mouth, medication can be given through the rectum by means of a _____, under the tongue _____, through patches on the skin, by injection into the skin, and through intravenous injections.

22. The home health aide's responsibilities in pain management include _____ and _____ the client in pain, and reporting when the pain medication ordered for the client is no longer _____.

23. List five comfort measures the home health aide can provide to the dying client.

    a. _____

    b. _____

    c. _____

    d. _____

    e. _____

24. Signs of approaching death include:

    a. _____

    b. _____

    c. _____

    d. _____

    e. _____

    f. _____

25. Death is a _____ _____ that calls for certain formalities. A health care provider must complete a _____ _____ that states the cause of death, and formally register the death.

26. In some cases, a death may have to be investigated by a medical examiner or

    _____.

27. An _____ is a detailed examination of the body to determine the cause of death and may provide more information about the client's illness. It may be requested by the family or by law in the event of an unexpected death.

28. List the duties of a home health aide when the client dies.

    a. _____

    b. _____

    c. _____

    d. _____

29. The client should be treated with _____ and _____ at all times.

30. It is important for the home health aide to remain _____ when death occurs.

31. A death that is sudden is more _____ than one following a long illness.

32. Religious practices differ from person to person, the aide needs to become _____ with the family and the client's practices.

33. _____ is treating the body with preservatives to prevent decay and is forbidden in Jewish religious practice.

34. The _____ _____ is the physical and emotional response to a loss, and the process of accepting it.

35. _____ is a private journey that is different for everyone, influenced by cultural and family differences. It needs to be expressed or processed, so it can be _____.

Matching. *Match each religion with beliefs and practices related to dying and death.*

36. ____ Judaism

37. ____ Roman Catholic

38. ____ Christian Scientist

39. ____ Muslim

40. ____ Hinduism

a. Autopsy permitted. Priest ties thread around neck or wrist and pours water in mouth. Only family and friends touch body.

b. Autopsy unlikely, organ donation not permitted. No ritual performed before or after death.

c. Autopsy permitted only for medical or legal reasons, no organ donation. No ritual before or after death.

d. Autopsy and organ donation permitted. Sacrament of the Sick administered to ill client or shortly after death.

e. Torah and Psalms read; no embalming; conversation kept to minimum; body not touched up to 30 minutes after death. Someone stays with the body until burial, usually within 24 hours. Mirrors may be covered at family's request.

True or False. *Answer the following statements true (T) or false (F).*

41. T   F   Some medical advances prolong life but do not improve life.

42. T   F   The home health aide should offer advice to the client or family of the dying client.

43. T   F   The unconscious client cannot hear what is being said.

44. T   F   Good communication skills are important when working with the dying client and family.

45. T   F   If grief is not expressed, symptoms or erratic behavior or failing health may appear.

Multiple Choice. *Choose the correct answer or answers.*

46. The last sense to be lost in a dying client is

   a. sight

   b. hearing

   c. touch

   d. smell

47. The hospice program accepts clients that generally have

   a. less than one year to live

   b. less than three months to live

   c. cancer

   d. six months to live

48. The five stages of dying were first described by

    a. Einstein

    b. Bill Clinton

    c. Dr. Elisabeth Kübler-Ross

    d. The Patient Self-Determination Act

49. The most difficult time for the family after the death of a loved one is

    a. the first two or three months

    b. from the third to sixth month

    c. from sixth to ninth month

    d. from the ninth to twelfth month

Documentation Exercises. *Read the following descriptions and provide documentation for each scenario.*

50. You have been caring for Mr. Howe for a week. He had a stroke and has been unconscious. You are aware that the health care provider thinks that he is not going to recover. His daughter greets you as you walk in to care for him. She tells you that he moves in his sleep and that she knows now that he will recover. You know that many times unconscious people move, but that particular movement is a neurological reaction. You want to reassure her, but you know that he is not expected to improve. What will you tell her? What do you document? What else should you do with this information?

51. When you arrive to care for Mr. Howe, you notice that he has noisy, labored respirations and his pulse is very weak and irregular. You feel that death is approaching. What do you document? What will you tell his relatives?

PRACTICE SITUATIONS

Case 1

You are caring for a terminal client, Mr. Montes. He is having problems accepting the fact that he is terminal. He keeps telling you about the plans he is making for next summer. He has even offered to take you fishing to a special spot where he knows you will be able to catch a big fish.

Questions

1. What stage of grieving is he in?

2. What can you do to help him accept the fact that he is dying?

3. How do you feel about working with him?

Case 2

When you arrive at the home of your client, you find him alone. When you approach him you notice that he is very still. You feel his wrist for a pulse, and his hand is cold. You cannot find a pulse. You place your head close to his chest and you cannot hear any signs of breathing.

Questions

1. What do you do first?

2. Do you need to call anyone? If so, who?

3. What about relatives?

4. You do not know whether he has any relatives nearby. How will you find out about this?

CROSSWORD PUZZLE

Across

1 final stage of a fatal illness

5 statement regarding end of life care

7 unconsciousness prior to death

8 person appointed to make decisions when client is unable to speak for himself or herself

9 program provides care for dying clients and family

Down

2 papers that specify the type of treatment clients do or do not want under serious medical conditions

3 physical and emotional response to a loss

4 care provided when no longer seeking a cure

6 discoloration of skin before death

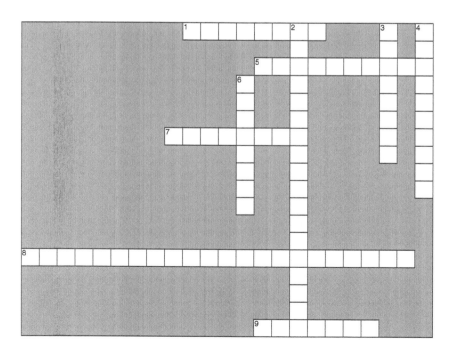

UNIT QUIZ

Short Answer/Fill in the Blanks. *Complete the following sentences with the correct word or words.*

1. Due to increased life expectancy with three and four generations living at the same time, _____ experiences in some families have been rare.

2. Persons who have been given a diagnosis that death will likely occur within the next six months may choose _____ _____.

3. Hospice program services are most often offered in the client's _____; some hospices provide services in the hospital or _____-_____ care facilities.

4. The goal of hospice is to assist the _____ and _____ to make the dying process as pain-free and comfortable as possible.

5. The criterion to enter a hospice program is that the client's _____ _____ is less than six months due to a _____ _____.

6. The final stage of a fatal illness is called the _____ _____.

7. Care given to a client who knows there is no cure for his or her illness, emphasizing quality of life and not prolonging death, is called _____ _____.

8. List five signs of approaching death.

   a. _____

   b. _____

   c. _____

   d. _____

   e. _____

9. Cultural and family differences will influence the death and dying process including the public behavior of _____.

10. The _____ _____ is the physical and emotional response to a loss, and the process of accepting the loss.

True or False. *Answer the following statements true (T) or false (F).*

11. T F The five stages of grief are normal reactions to help people deal with approaching death.

12. T F If you are uncomfortable with a dying client, you should not say anything to your agency because you need your job.

13. T F One of the duties of the home health aide is to notify the health care provider at the time of the client's death.

14. T F A client who is terminally ill is unlikely to recover.

15. T F If a client is angry with you and says, "Why get dressed? I'm going to die anyway," you should view this as a normal reaction.

16. T F Listening to a family regarding the care of the client is one of the duties of the home health aide.

17. T F Postmortem care is care provided when a client dies.

18. T F Comatose is a state of unconsciousness just before death.

19. T F It is not important for the home health aide to keep the nurse informed on the status of the client or any changes occurring, as the nurse will observe them on the next visit.

Matching. *Match each stage of grief with a statement about the stage.*

20. ____ denial

21. ____ anger

22. ____ bargaining

23. ____ depression

24. ____ acceptance

a. calmly facing what is to be or feeling a sense of peace

b. "Dear God, I'll be good. Please not yet."

c. "This can't be happening to me."

d. feeling that this death is unfair; bitterness

e. brooding, withdrawal, "I cannot go on living."

Multiple Choice. *Choose the correct answer or answers.*

25. The hospice care involves a team of professionals including
    a. health care providers and nurses
    b. home health aides
    c. clergy and volunteers
    d. all of the above

26. The hospice team helps with
    a. pain management and comfort care
    b. social and financial concerns
    c. spiritual concerns
    d. all of the above

27. In 1991, a law was passed requiring home health agencies receiving Medicare and Medicaid to implement procedures to increase public awareness regarding the rights of clients to make choices about health care. This is called the
    a. advanced directives
    b. Patient Self-Determination Act
    c. living will
    d. Hospice Care Act

28. Papers that specify the type of treatment clients want or do not want under serious medical conditions, in which they may be unable to communicate their wishes to a health care provider or family, is called
    a. advanced directives
    b. durable power of attorney
    c. living will
    d. last acts

29. Treating the body with preservatives after death to prevent decay is called
    a. embalming
    b. rigor mortis
    c. mottling
    d. autopsy

30. A detailed examination of the body to determine the exact cause of death is called an
    a. embalming
    b. rigor mortis
    c. mottling
    d. autopsy

31. Examples of religious and cultural differences influencing the death and dying process include all but

    a. Native Americans and Inuit people used to leave their loved ones alone to die.

    b. Among some Jewish families, burial occurs within 24 hours, embalming is forbidden, and the casket remains closed.

    c. Baptist clergy ministers through counseling and prayers. Caskets are usually open, with some faces covered with a handkerchief.

    d. All clients' bodies are washed after death.

32. The home health aide's responsibilities in caring for the dying client include

    a. Creating and maintaining a trusting relationship with the client.

    b. Observing and monitoring the client for pain, including reporting when the pain medication ordered for the client appears to be no longer effective.

    c. Reporting how the client is handling the emotional stress of the terminal illness.

    d. Providing comfort measures.

    e. All of the above.

33. The nursing supervisor informs you that Mrs. Embers is dying. Signs you may see include

    a. noisy, irregular respirations

    b. cool, moist, and clammy skin

    c. body relaxes and jaw drops

    d. incontinence of bowel and bladder

    e. all of the above

34. Comfort measures the home health aide may provide include all but

    a. changing client position every two hours

    b. providing mouth care every two hours along with lip moisturizer

    c. administering pain medications with sips of water

    d. instilling artificial eyedrops, as eye blinking may cease

35. Additional activities the home health aide can do to promote a soothing atmosphere in the home include all except

    a. holding the client's hand

    b. providing bright lights or sunshine

    c. playing soft music

    d. reading from the Bible or other books

36. Mr. Kemp was diagnosed with end-stage liver cancer two months ago. His skin is yellow and his abdomen is very large. As you arrive in the home, he starts yelling, "What good am I . . . I hate what's happened to my body" and angrily glares at you. What response should the aide make?

    a. "I don't need to listen to you yell at me."

    b. "Mr. Kemp, it sounds like you are upset and angry, I'm here to listen if you want to talk."

    c. Call the nursing supervisor and tell her you are leaving because the client is yelling at you.

    d. "Mr. Kemp, stop this type of talk right now."

37. Mr. Kemp's legs become very pale. Discoloration of the skin is noted, especially on the back. This is called

    a. embalming

    c. mottling

    b. rigor mortis

    d. autopsy

38. During your next visit with Mr. Kemp, he stops breathing. You should

    a. Write down the time of death.

    b. Call the case manager immediately, who will contact the health care provider.

    c. Call a family member, if none present, after the health care provider has been notified of the death.

    d. Follow the case manager's instructions and clean the client's body.

    e. All of the above.

39. You attend Mr. Kemp's funeral. Some family members are sitting quietly in a corner talking, while his wife is visibly sobbing as she greets each mourner. Your understanding of the grieving process is

    a. Grief is an individual experience, with various ways to express oneself.

    b. As people work through their emotions, they come to accept the loss.

    c. The grief process can take a long time and it is hard work.

    d. If grief is not expressed, symptoms of erratic behavior or failing health may appear.

    e. All of the above.

UNIT 22   CARING FOR THE CLIENT WITH ALZHEIMER'S DISEASE

LEARNING OBJECTIVES

After studying this unit, you should be able to:
- Describe the term *dementia*
- Discuss how Alzheimer's disease is diagnosed
- List the 10 warning signs of Alzheimer's disease
- Discuss the five stages of Alzheimer's disease
- Discuss the various behaviors that are characteristic of Alzheimer's disease
- Discuss how to work with clients who display various behaviors such as wandering and sundowning
- Identify the benefits of using habilitation, validation therapy, and reminiscence when working with clients with dementia
- List five tips for communicating with the client with dementia

TERMS TO DEFINE

- Alzheimer's disease
- catastrophic behavior
- dementia
- habilitation
- hoarding
- pillaging
- reality orientation
- reminiscence
- repetitive behaviors
- Safe Return Home Program
- shadowing
- sundowning
- suspiciousness
- validation therapy
- wandering

APPLICATION EXERCISES

Short Answer/Fill in the Blanks. *Complete the following sentences with the correct word or words.*

1. Dementia is characterized by _____ _____
   _____, with Alzheimer's disease being the most common form.

2. The client with dementia will experience impaired _____, inability to
   _____, along with loss of _____, reasoning ability, and loss of judgment.

3. Risk factors for Alzheimer's disease are being female, Black ethnicity, having
   _____ _____ _____, family history, and old
   age: the disease strikes _____% of people over age 65 and
   _____% of people over age 85.

4. Five signs and symptoms of Alzheimer's disease are:

   a. _____

   b. _____

   c. _____

   d. _____

   e. _____

5. List 10 warning signs of Alzheimer's disease.

   a. _____

   b. _____

   c. _____

   d. _____

   e. _____

   f. _____

   g. _____

   h. _____

   i. _____

   j. _____

6. The home health aide caring for an Alzheimer's client must have a great deal of
   _____, _____, and _____ of the disease
   process.

7. If the client becomes upset about something, try to _____ him or her with
   something else.

8. The family caring for a relative with Alzheimer's disease needs to have times of
   _____ away from the client.

9. Four things the home health aide can do to assist the client in communication are:

   a. _____

   b. _____

   c. _____

   d. _____

10. A client with Alzheimer's disease should be taken to the bathroom every
    _____ hours.

11. The home health aide should be aware of possible side effects of any _____
    the client is taking.

12. If the client exhibits disruptive behavior, the home health aide should try to determine the
    _____ of the behavior.

13. Validation therapy is used to increase _____ and _____ the
    client's feelings.

14. These clients have little short-term memory, but many _____ memories remain.

15. Exploring memories of the past with the client is called _____.

16. List five tips for clients with changes in eating patterns to help improve nutrition.

    a. _____

    b. _____

    c. _____

    d. _____

    e. _____

True or False. *Answer the following statements true (T) or false (F).*

17. T F Alzheimer's disease is the third leading cause of death in the adult population.

18. T F The time from onset to death can range from 3 to 20 years in Alzheimer's disease.

19. T F There is a specific test for Alzheimer's disease.

20. T F If you forget the food cooking on the stove, you probably have Alzheimer's disease.

21. T F Consistency is extremely important when caring for clients with Alzheimer's disease.

22. T F Clients with Alzheimer's disease cannot control their behavior.

23. T F The client with Alzheimer's disease sleeps for many hours without interruption.

24. T F Playing soft, soothing music helps calm the agitated client.

25. T F Wandering is the most common agitated behavior among clients with Alzheimer's disease.

Matching. *Match the stage of dementia with the level of impairment.*

26. ____ body functions slowly shut down, client says about six words

27. ____ client experiences some memory problems but is able to live independently

28. ____ client experiences severe problems communicating, requires caregiver to perform activities of daily living

29. ____ severe memory loss occurs; behaviors such as wandering, sleeplessness, and shadowing are evident

30. ____ short lapses of memory occur and client has problems with everyday thinking skills

a. mild cognitive impairment

b. mild dementia

c. moderate dementia

d. severe dementia

e. profound dementia

Multiple Choice. *Choose the correct answer or answers.*

31. Alzheimer's disease is identified by
    a. a blood test
    b. documentation of behaviors and symptoms over time
    c. an x-ray of the skull
    d. all of these

32. The home health aide caring for an Alzheimer's client needs
    a. patience
    b. understanding of the symptoms
    c. to know the client cannot help his or her behavior
    d. all of these

33. If the client has difficulty walking, the aide can
    a. remove scatter rugs   c. a and b
    b. pick up small objects on the floor   d. none of these

34. One way to prevent the client from wandering is to
    a. keep the client locked in a room
    b. keep the doors locked leading to the outside of home
    c. tell the client that his or her behavior is inappropriate
    d. place large-print signs on doors "DO NOT GO OUT" or "TURN AROUND"

35. Ways to assist the client experiencing dementia are all but
    a. scolding or punishing the client for this behavior
    b. encouraging fluids as usual till early evening to prevent dehydration
    c. use simple, washable clothing with Velcro-type tabs to help get garments on and off easier
    d. provide visual cues: signs on door, picture of toilet, and leave night-light on

36. A response to stimuli that is overwhelming to the client is called
    a. sundowning   c. repetitive behaviors
    b. suspiciousness   d. catastrophic behavior

37. Catastrophic behavior involves
    a. the client collecting and putting things away in a special place
    b. client taking things or items belonging to someone else and insisting they are his or her own
    c. client screaming, cursing, threatening, hitting, or biting due to being overwhelmed
    d. following the caregiver around and mimicking the behavior of others

38. The home health aide can assist the client with catastrophic behavior by

    a. asking the family or other caregiver for ideas on how to approach the client

    b. noting what appears to trigger these behaviors and involving the client in situations less likely to trigger these behaviors

    c. avoiding trying to reason with the client when he or she is having one of these attacks

    d. all of the above

    e. none of the above

39. Repetitive behaviors are seen often in dementia: repeating the same question, phrase, story, or activity repeatedly. What can be done to help relieve caregiver burden and prevent burnout?

    a. have the client participate in adult day care

    b. encourage caregiver to join a support group

    c. recommend that the main caregiver take time off at definite intervals, with the home health aide providing respite care

    d. all of the above

    e. none of the above

40. The home health aide's responsibilities in medication management include all but

    a. being responsible for administering medications on time

    b. monitoring the time, dose, and side effects of the client's medication

    c. being aware of the client's medication schedule and reminding the client to take prepoured doses

    d. reporting to the nurse or case manager any medication side effects suspected, or refusal or spitting out of medications

Documentation Exercises. *Read the following descriptions and provide documentation for each scenario.*

41. When you arrive at the home of Mrs. Lee, she runs out the door past you. You know that her diagnosis is Alzheimer's disease and that she likes to wander around the neighborhood. It is very cold outside, and she is dressed only in a nightgown. Document your interventions.

42. After you have dressed Mrs. Lee and taken her for a walk, you try to feed her. She spits the food at you. You know that this is typical behavior for Mrs. Lee, so you blend the food and give it to her as a shake, which she drinks. Document your care activities.

PRACTICE SITUATIONS

Case 1

Your client is diagnosed with Alzheimer's disease. He is easily distracted, and you have had increasing problems caring for him. When you are bathing him, he walks out of the shower and runs out the door. When you are helping him eat, he stands suddenly, knocking the food all over the floor.

Questions

1. What can you do to modify these problems?

2. Is there any way to alter his behavior?

Case 2

You have been working with Mr. Kai for several weeks. At a recent case conference, the team decided to try reminiscence with him.

Questions

1. Describe reminiscence therapy.

2. What will your role in this therapy be?

3. Why is it successful with the elderly?

CROSSWORD PUZZLE

Across

1 collecting and putting items in a special place

9 technique to increase self-esteem and validate client's feelings when client remains in the past

10 loss of mind

11 behavior changes occurring in late afternoon and evening

12 most common form of dementia

Down

2 recalling memories by reviewing life history

3 stimulus response when overwhelmed

4 taking things belonging to someone else but insisting and thinking they are his or her own

5 care focuses on what the client can do, not what the client used to do

6 client repeats same words or actions repeatedly

7 most common agitated behavior

8 client follows and mimics behavior

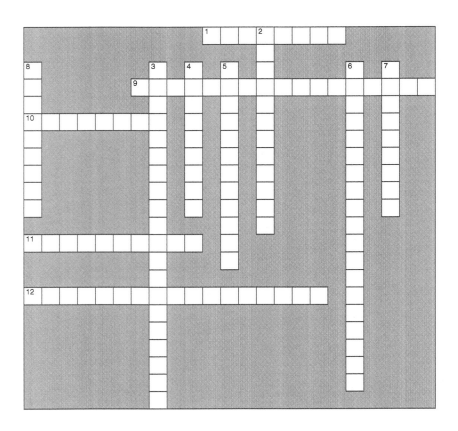

UNIT QUIZ

Short Answer/Fill in the Blanks. *Complete the following sentences with the correct word or words.*

1. Progressive mental deterioration or loss of mind is called _____.

2. Clients with dementia experience impaired _____, inability to _____, _____ of memory along with loss of reasoning ability and _____.

3. Five warning signs of Alzheimer's disease are:

   a. _____

   b. _____

   c. _____

   d. _____

   e. _____

4. List a client's experience that occurs with each stage of dementia.

   a. mild cognitive impairment: _____

   b. mild dementia: _____

   c. moderate dementia: _____

   d. severe dementia: _____

   e. profound dementia: _____

5. _____ _____ is a response to stimuli that is overwhelming with the client screaming, cursing, threatening, hitting, or biting as a result.

6. Support groups help _____ _____ meet to share common problems, learn how to cope better with their parent or relative, as well as face up to their own feelings or fears.

7. Therapy interventions used to help a client with dementia include: _____ therapy, _____ and _____ orientation.

8. List five guidelines for keeping the home environment safe.

   a. _____

   b. _____

   c. _____

   d. _____

   e. _____

9. The most common agitated behavior among people with Alzheimer's disease is _____.

10. List five responsibilities the home health aide has in caring for clients with Alzheimer's disease.

a. _____

b. _____

c. _____

d. _____

e. _____

Matching. *Match each term with the behavior or therapy.*

11. ____ sundowning

12. ____ wandering

13. ____ suspiciousness

14. ____ hoarding

15. ____ catastrophic behavior

16. ____ shadowing

17. ____ pillaging

18. ____ repetitive behaviors

19. ____ validation therapy

20. ____ reminiscence

a. most common agitated behavior

b. behavior in the late afternoon and evening

c. screaming, cursing, threatening, hitting, biting

d. accuses caregiver and others of stealing items

e. client collects and puts things in special place

f. takes things or items belonging to others

g. follows caregiver around and mimics behaviors

h. repeats same question, story, and activity repeatedly

i. memories recalled, reviewing life history

j. communication technique to increase self-esteem and validate client's feelings

Multiple Choice. *Choose the correct answer or answers.*

21. A symptom of Alzheimer's disease is

a. gradual memory loss

b. disorientation

c. personality changes

d. loss of language skills

e. all of these

22. All of the following are causes of wandering except

a. The client is looking for something.

b. It is a remedy for pain and suffering.

c. The client is looking for a place to lie down.

d. The client wants to exercise his or her legs.

23. Which therapy's purpose is to recall long-term and deep-seated memories by reviewing past life history?

    a. validation

    b. reminiscence

    c. reality orientation

    d. habilitation

24. The term used to describe care for the client, which focuses on what the client can do, not what the client used to do is called

    a. validation

    b. reminiscence

    c. reality orientation

    d. habilitation

25. In clients with mild to moderate memory loss and for those who understand simple words, simple memory aids such as prominent calendar, list of daily tasks, clocks, signs, and family members photos can help orient the client to the present. This is called

    a. validation

    b. reminiscence

    c. reality orientation

    d. habilitation

26. An Alzheimer's client who is confused, frightened, or in pain might demonstrate behavior that is troublesome. What can the aide do to assist the client?

    a. Tell the client to "get his or her act together."

    b. Note what appears to trigger the behavior and take steps to minimize these situations in the future.

    c. Protect the client from self-injury.

    d. Request that the family medicate the client.

27. Mr. Anderson often is observed with the sundowning behavior of pacing at nighttime. All except one of the following actions can help decrease this behavior.

    a. Promote resting in bed during the morning.

    b. Keep the client reasonably busy with activities during the day.

    c. Offer rest periods between activities, but discourage sleeping in bed.

    d. Provide an enclosed area for the client to take walks in the daytime.

28. "My sister Suzy took my green pants," Mr. Anderson yells one day as you enter his room. You see him rummaging through his dresser drawers. The best response to make is

    a. "Let's look in the laundry room for them," and distract him after leaving the bedroom.

    b. Ask Suzy if she saw the pants, and tear the house apart looking for them.

    c. "I like you in your blue pants best."

    d. "Suzy threw the pants out because the seam was ripped."

29. You are scheduled to cook lunch for Mrs. Gleason, a new client who has arthritis. Looking in her refrigerator, you see that an ice cream container on the refrigerator shelf is leaking. A check of the freezer finds a box of cereal, a sugar bowl, and a frozen, opened milk container. You suspect that Mrs. Gleason has

    a. mild dementia

    b. moderate dementia

    c. severe dementia

    d. profound dementia

30. What should be done with your observations of Mrs. Gleason's refrigerator?

    a. Document your findings in home health aide notes.

    b. Call the client's nurse or clinical manager and report the findings.

    c. Call 911.

    d. Do nothing, as it's none of your business.

31. You have cared for Mr. Petry, a client with mild dementia, for three months. Mrs. Petry confides to you on your next visit to the home that her husband left home to take a walk, got lost, couldn't remember his home address, and was brought home by the police. What safety advice should you offer her?

    a. Recommend that Mr. Petry wear a Medic Alert bracelet listing his name, address, phone number, and medical condition.

    b. Have a picture taken of him for ease of identity in case he leaves home, and place his name inside of his clothes.

    c. Notify police and fire departments of his condition, along with registering with the Safe Return Home Program.

    d. Keep outside doors locked and signs posted such as "DO NOT GO OUT."

    e. All of the above.

32. The benefits of medications used to treat clients with dementia include all but

    a. slowing the progression of illness

    b. soothing agitation and anxiety

    c. promoting sleeplessness

    d. enhancing the client's ability to participate in activities

33. Important safety tips for the client who has difficulty walking include all but

    a. picking up and putting away objects the client may not see and trip over such as small footstools, doorstops, plants, and pet toys

    b. keeping floors polished and waxed

    c. making sure the client's shoes fit properly

    d. encouraging clients to sit only in chairs with arms

34. Mr. Lightfoot exhibits restlessness and agitation in late afternoon. Which home health aide actions would not help decrease this behavior?

    a. Decrease the level of activity in late afternoon to reduce potential stress.

    b. Play soft, soothing music or distract the client with quiet, simple activities.

    c. Try to reason the client out of his behavior.

    d. Apply restraints if the behavior escalates.

35. Ways to promote bathing and oral hygiene with Miss Tyler include all but

    a. Organize all the necessary equipment before you bring the client to the bathroom.

    b. Ensure the client's safety when bathing: use handholds, nonslip mats, and tub seats.

    c. Sponge baths can be effective intermittently, but insist on a weekly shower or tub bath to ensure proper cleansing of all skin surfaces.

    d. Make the client feel in control: involve and coach the client by suggesting steps if necessary

36. Mr. Robinson exhibits improper sexual behavior at times by fondling himself during bath or dropping his pants in the hallway. What actions should the home health aide take?

    a. Try reasoning with the client regarding his behavior.

    b. Scold the client for his inappropriate behavior.

    c. Do not over react, remain calm. If the client is in public when dropping his pants, quickly pull up his pants and remove him from the scene.

    d. Provide appropriate touching to show that you care for and value the client.

37. An association that can link families with resources in their community to help them cope with this disease is the

    a. Alzheimer's Association

    b. National Dementia Society

    c. Support Groups International

    d. American Association of Retired Persons

UNIT 23 CARING FOR THE CLIENT WITH CANCER

LEARNING OBJECTIVES

After studying this unit, you should be able to:
- Define benign, malignant, metastasis, and carcinogens
- List seven warning signs of cancer
- List four screening tests for cancer
- Name three ways cancer can be treated
- List precautions to use when caring for a client receiving chemotherapy and radiation therapy
- List four common side effects from cancer therapy
- Discuss breast and testicular self-examination
- Describe the nursing care given to a client with cancer
- Describe the appearance of a cancerous skin lesion

TERMS TO DEFINE

- abdominal perineal resection
- benign
- benign prostatic hypertrophy (BPH)
- biopsy
- cachexia
- cancer
- carcinogen
- chemotherapy
- colonoscopy
- encapsulated
- hysterectomy
- laryngectomy
- larynx
- lobectomy
- lumpectomy
- malignant
- mammogram
- mastectomy
- melanoma
- metastasis
- panhysterectomy
- pneumonectomy
- prostate-specific antigen (PSA)
- prosthesis
- remission
- sigmoidoscopy
- stoma
- trachea
- tracheostomy
- transurethral resection of the prostate (TURP)

APPLICATION EXERCISES

Short Answer/Fill in the Blanks. *Complete the following sentences with the correct word or words.*

1. An uncontrolled growth of abnormal cells is called _____.

2. Cancer cells steal _____ from surrounding cells and push _____ cells out of the way.

3. Cancer cells cause changes in the body, producing _____ that indicate something is wrong.

4. The seven warning signs of cancer are:

   a. _____

   b. _____

   c. _____

   d. _____

   e. _____

   f. _____

   g. _____

5. A _____ is a substance or agent that produces cancer; the general group includes _____, environmental factors, hormones, and viruses.

6. The process in which some cancerous cells break away from the original tumor and move to other parts of the body is called _____.

7. When cancer is treated and does not reappear for five years, the cancer is considered cured or in _____.

8. Each day, more than _____ people die from some form of cancer. There are more than _____ types of cancer.

9. A _____, or sample, of body tissue is done if the health care provider suspects an individual has cancer. This is done to confirm the diagnosis and find out what _____ of cancer the tumor is.

10. Three cancers that occur most often in women are:

    a. _____

    b. _____

    c. _____

11. Name three cancers that occur most often in men.

    a. _____

    b. _____

    c. _____

12. Treatment of cancer includes _____, _____, and _____.

13. Rays aimed deep into the body to reach cancer cells and destroy them are called _____.

14. Clients undergoing radiation therapy will have their treatment areas outlined in
_____ _____ or may even be outlined in tiny tattoos.

15. List five side effects of chemotherapy and radiation.

a. _____

b. _____

c. _____

d. _____

e. _____

16. Precautions the home health aide should take for 48 hours after a client has received chemotherapy treatment include:

a. _____

b. _____

c. _____

17. The client with cancer needs to have a diet high in _____ and
_____ to prevent malnutrition and _____ to prevent dehydration.

18. The terminal cancer client may have a distinctive _____ due to the death of body cells and may require a room _____.

19. The goal of cancer therapy in the final stages is to keep the client _____ and with the least amount of _____.

20. The dying client may be admitted to _____ care.

21. All women should have a yearly _____ to test for cancer of the
_____.

22. If the female has cancer of the uterus, a _____ may be necessary.

23. After a mastectomy, the client needs to follow the _____ program started at the hospital; the home health aide can help the client with this.

24. A free service provided by the American Cancer Society available to the postmastectomy client is called _____ _____ _____
_____.

25. After mastectomy, a _____ may be made for the client.

26. Several illnesses affecting the respiratory system are _____,
_____, and _____.

27. Five signs of lung cancer are:

a. _____

b. _____

c. _____

d. _____

e. _____

28. Removal of part of the lung is called _____.

29. The client with lung cancer may require _____ therapy.

30. If the client has trouble breathing when lying down, many _____ should be offered.

31. The trachea is the airway between the nasal passages and the _____.

32. The part of the trachea called the voice box is the _____.

33. A treatment for cancer of the larynx is removal of the larynx, or _____.

34. A surgical opening into the trachea is called a _____.

35. The dressing over the tracheostomy stoma should be kept _____ to avoid inhaling dust.

36. Speech therapists work with the client after a _____ to help the client to learn to speak again.

37. The home health aide needs to be alert to any _____ or _____ _____ from the tracheostomy.

True or False. *Answer the following statements true (T) or false (F).*

38. T   F   The exact cause of cancer is unknown.

39. T   F   Carcinogens can be chemical, environmental factors, hormones, or viruses.

40. T   F   Cancer is the leading cause of death each year.

41. T   F   A hysterectomy inhibits the enjoyment of sex for the woman.

42. T   F   Fibroid tumors of the uterus are not cancerous.

43. T   F   After hysterectomy, hormones are given to the female clients to replace those normally produced.

44. T   F   There has been an increase in cancer of the colon and stomach each year.

45. T   F   If a woman notices a lump in her breast, she can wait until her next regularly scheduled appointment to tell her health care provider.

46. T   F   It is important for a woman to have the support of her family after undergoing a mastectomy.

47. T   F   Only lung cancer exceeds colon cancer in the number of new cases and deaths each year.

Matching. *Match each term with the correct definition.*

48. _____ carcinogen
49. _____ malignant
50. _____ benign
51. _____ biopsy
52. _____ remission
53. _____ metastasis
54. _____ mammogram
55. _____ mastectomy
56. _____ hysterectomy
57. _____ chemotherapy

a. noncancerous

b. no longer growing

c. surgical removal of the uterus

d. use of chemicals to attack cancer

e. sample of tissue from the area with cellular changes

f. x-ray of breast

g. cancerous

h. cancer producing

i. surgical removal of breast

j. spreading of the cancer to other tissues

Multiple Choice. *Choose the correct answer or answers.*

58. Diets for clients with cancer are usually

    a. low calorie

    c. high calorie, high protein

    b. semiliquid

    d. high fiber

59. It is important for women to perform breast self-examinations

    a. once a week

    b. once a year

    c. once a month

    d. only if they choose not to see a health care provider every year

60. Breast self-examination procedure

    a. should be done 7 to 10 days after each period

    b. involves checking each breast for changes in shape, swelling, nipple discharge

    c. is performed lying down with finger pads of three middle fingers firmly pressed on breast moving in circular or up and down pattern; repeat standing up

    d. all of the above

61. The purpose of a Pap smear test is to

    a. detect early skin cancer

    b. detect early cellular changes in the uterus

    c. detect early cellular changes in the cervix

    d. be used in place of a biopsy

62. Prostate cancer tests include

    a. prostate-specific antigen (PSA)

    b. Pap smear

    c. colonoscopy

    d. digital rectal exam by health care provider

63. Advanced prostate cancer signs include

    a. frequency of urination

    c. decrease in size and force of stream

    b. urinary retention

    d. burning on urination

64. Surgery indicated for benign prostatic hypertrophy is called

    a. transurethral resection of the prostate (TURP)

    b. hysterectomy

    c. urinary catheterization

    d. prostatectomy

65. Signs of lung cancer include

    a. constant vomiting, earache

    c. coughing up blood, chest pain

    b. persistent hacking cough

    d. none of these

66. A tracheostomy is
    a. performed as part of cancer of larynx treatment
    b. a surgical opening made into the trachea below the larynx
    c. an artificial airway that can be used to supply oxygen to the lungs
    d. all of the above

67. Skin cancer is most often caused by excessive exposure to
    a. sunlight and sunburn
    b. harsh chemicals
    c. tanning booths
    d. excessive vitamin use

Documentation Exercises. *Read the following descriptions and provide documentation for each scenario.*

68. You are caring for Mrs. Plum. She is recovering from a mastectomy. She is weeping and very upset. She is convinced that she is going to die, even though the health care provider has informed her that the tumor was very small and the chances of it reoccurring are very slight. Mrs. Plum's family is very supportive of her. How will you reassure her? What can you tell her relatives? Document your care.

69. You are assigned to care for Mr. Ken. He has just returned from the hospital, where he received a chemotherapy treatment. He feels very fatigued. He sometimes becomes nauseated after chemotherapy. What precautions do you need to take? He tells you that he is not hungry. What can you do to encourage Mr. Ken to eat?

PRACTICE SITUATIONS

Case 1

Your client, Mrs. Jonas, has been undergoing a course of chemotherapy. She has lost 20 pounds and is very thin. She is nauseated all the time. She feels very discouraged at times; she has told you that she thinks the chemotherapy will kill her before the cancer does.

Questions

1. What can you do to improve her appetite?
2. Can you think of anything to tell her that will make her less discouraged?
3. Will these problems continue after her therapy is finished?

Case 2

Your client, Mrs. Polaski, has recently been diagnosed with cancer. Her physician has explained the options to her. She has decided not to have chemotherapy or surgery. She has heard of an alternate cure for cancer. It involves taking up to 100 vitamin pills a day. You feel that the treatment she has chosen will not be successful.

Questions

1. What should you do with this information?
2. You know that she has the right to choose her treatment, but you are concerned that she has not chosen the correct treatment. How will you cope with your feelings?

CROSSWORD PUZZLE

Across

3 malignant skin cancer

6 surgical opening into the trachea

7 no longer growing or spreading

8 drugs used to treat cancer

12 noncancerous tumor stays in one area

13 blood test to screen for prostate cancer

14 marked wasting of the body

15 surgical removal of breast tissue

Down

1 substance or agent that produces cancer

2 transurethral resection of the prostate

4 x-ray to detect breast cancer

5 sample of body tissue

8 uncontrolled growth of abnormal cells

9 spreading of cancer to other body tissues

10 surgical removal of uterus and cervix

11 artificial breast

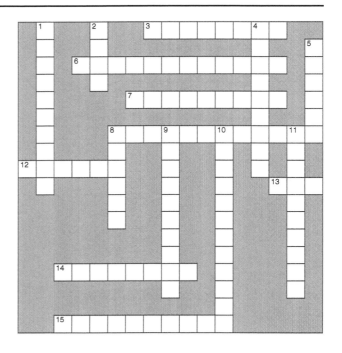

UNIT QUIZ

Short Answer/Fill in the Blanks. *Complete the following sentences with the correct word or words.*

1. Cancer is the uncontrolled growth of _____.

2. A substance or agent that produces cancer is called a _____.

3. The _____ cancer is detected, the less chance it has of _____ to other parts of the body.

4. A _____ tumor tends to be encapsulated or confined to an area while _____ tumor cells spread rapidly and infiltrate other areas of the body.

5. The spread of cancer to other body tissues is called _____.

6. Three treatments for cancer include _____, _____, and _____.

7. List four tests to detect cancer.

   a. _____

   b. _____

   c. _____

   d. _____

8. Five signs of colon cancer are:

   a. _____

   b. _____

   c. _____

   d. _____

   e. _____

9. The first sign of skin cancer is a _____ on the skin that does not _____.

10. List five things the home health aide can do to improve nutrition for the cancer client.

   a. _____

   b. _____

   c. _____

   d. _____

   e. _____

True or False. *Answer the following statements true (T) or false (F).*

11. T F   The goal of cancer therapy in the final stages is to keep the client as comfortable as possible with the least amount of pain.

12. T F   A lump found in the breast during self-examination will probably be malignant.

13. T F   A hysterectomy is the removal of the fallopian tubes, ovaries, uterus, and cervix.

14. T F   The American Cancer Society's Reach to Recovery program is a free service to meet the physical, emotional, and cosmetic needs of women with breast cancer.

15. T F   Only older men need to perform testicular self-exam.

16. T F   Lung cancer signs include persistent hoarseness, sudden weight loss, shortness of breath, or coughing up blood.

17. T F   Tracheostomy is surgical removal of the larynx.

18. T F   Speech therapy is important to help the laryngectomy client learn how to talk.

19. T F   It is important for the home health aide to assist the nurse in monitoring pain.

20. T F   Common types of skin cancer are basal cell and squamous cell.

Matching. *Match each term with the correct definition.*

21. ____ benign
22. ____ biopsy
23. ____ cancer
24. ____ chemotherapy
25. ____ hysterectomy
26. ____ malignant
27. ____ melanoma
28. ____ metastasis
29. ____ prosthesis
30. ____ stoma

a. surgical removal of the uterus and cervix
b. malignant skin cancer
c. surgical opening into the body
d. spreading of cancer to other tissues
e. noncancerous
f. tissue sample cut from area with cell changes
g. artificial breast
h. use of chemicals to attack cancer
i. cancerous tumors
j. uncontrolled growth of abnormal cells

Multiple Choice. *Choose the correct answer or answers.*

31. All of the following are warning signs of cancer except
    a. a change in bowel or bladder habits
    b. a lump or thickening in the breast or elsewhere in the body
    c. an obvious change in a wart or mole
    d. forgetfulness, memory loss, and blurred vision

32. Cancer can be treated by
    a. surgery
    b. radiotherapy
    c. chemotherapy
    d. all of the above

33. Chemotherapy and radiation side effects include
    a. nausea and vomiting, sore mouth and throat
    b. hair loss
    c. increased susceptibility to infections
    d. all of the above

34. Precautions for clients undergoing chemotherapy include all but
    a. Wash hands often.
    b. Do not use a hard toothbrush or floss teeth.
    c. Wear gloves for 48 hours after treatment when handling body fluids, soiled linens, or clothing,
    d. Wear mask, isolation gown, and goggles for all client contacts.

35. Guidelines for clients undergoing active cancer treatment include
    a. Avoid foods and juices high in acid content: tomato, orange, or grapefruit juice.
    b. Avoid salty or spicy foods.

c. Avoid commercial mouthwashes; rinse mouth with 1 teaspoon of baking soda mixed with warm water, holding rinse in mouth for about a minute.

d. All of the above.

36. The most common cancers in women are all but

a. thyroid

b. breast

c. colon

d. rectum

37. Miss Longbow was diagnosed with breast cancer and underwent a right-side modified mastectomy. What should the home health aide do to care for the client?

a. only take blood pressure on left arm

b. only take blood pressure on right arm

c. encourage client to exercise affected arm

d. all of the above

38. All of the following are concerns after breast cancer surgery except for

a. change in self-image

b. period of depression experienced

c. changes in bowel habits

d. need for support of loved ones

39. Testicular self-exam should be performed

a. starting as a young adult

b. after shower or bath when scrotum is relaxed

c. by holding the testicle between the thumbs and fingers with both hands and rolling it gently between the fingers, checking for lumps, pain, change in size

d. all of the above

40. Skin cancer screening includes reporting these changes to your health care provider

a. a change in color of a mole, especially black

b. change in shape or texture of mole

c. a mole that rises in height

d. all of the above

41. Mr. Peter has experienced unexplained anemia, fatigue, and change in bowel habits. These are signs of

a. colon cancer

b. breast cancer

c. rectal cancer

d. prostate cancer

42. Which of the following tests will the doctors perform to diagnose Mr. Peter's condition?

a. three stool specimens for hidden blood in stool

b. sigmoidoscopy

c. colostomy

d. Fleet enema

43. Mrs. Coleman was a heavy smoker. She has a raspy, hoarse voice, sudden weight loss, repeated bouts of bronchitis, and shortness of breath. You suspect she has

    a. breast cancer

    b. uterine cancer

    c. lung cancer

    d. skin cancer

44. The health care provider has informed her she will need a bronchoscopy and biopsy to determine if she has lung cancer. The biopsy report is positive and she is scheduled to undergo a lobectomy. This is

    a. removal of larynx

    b. removal of part of lung

    c. surgical opening into the trachea

    d. insertion of a small tube into trachea

45. Clients with lung cancer

    a. are cared for at home

    b. are transferred to hospice programs

    c. often need oxygen

    d. most likely will sit in a chair to breathe

46. Which of the following concerns about Mrs. Coleman should be reported to the nurse?

    a. client wearing oxygen cannula at 2 liters

    b. increasing shortness of breath

    c. bluishness of nails and lips

    d. need to use three pillows in bed

47. Mr. Wright has been having increasing trips to the bathroom, decreased urine stream, and feeling of urgency. He is experiencing signs of

    a. enlarged prostate

    b. urinary retention

    c. bowel cancer

    d. cervical cancer

48. Surgery is indicated for removal of the prostate and is called

    a. lobectomy

    b. hysterectomy

    c. colostomy

    d. transurethral resection of the prostate (TURP)

49. A common problem after TURP surgery is

    a. problems controlling the urine

    b. need to wear adult briefs until control is regained

    c. need to go to the bathroom every two hours

    d. all of the above

50. The home health aide can assist clients with cancer by

    a. providing high-calorie, protein-rich meals, and encouraging large amounts of fluids

    b. allowing the client to vent his or her emotions, with the aide responding using a nonjudgmental attitude

    c. space activities with rest periods to avoid extreme fatigue in client

    d. all of the above

SECTION 7
Maternal/Infant Care

UNIT 24   MATERNAL CARE

LEARNING OBJECTIVES

After studying this unit, you should be able to:
- List common pregnancy discomforts and their treatments
- Identify four high-risk pregnancies
- Recognize danger signals in pregnancy
- Explain the home health aide's responsibilities in caring for an expectant mother
- List common postpartum discomforts and their treatments
- Recognize postpartum abnormalities

TERMS TO DEFINE

- breast engorgement
- Down syndrome
- edema
- engagement
- fetal alcohol syndrome (FAS)
- flatulence
- heartburn
- hemorrhoids
- high-risk pregnancy
- lochia
- postpartum
- postpartum blues
- prenatal
- toxemia
- ultrasound
- varicose veins

APPLICATION EXERCISES

Short Answer/Fill in the Blanks. *Complete the following sentences with the correct word or words.*

1. A woman should seek medical care when she thinks she might be _____.
2. Frequent urination is due to the enlarged _____ sitting on the bladder.
3. The uterus dropping into the pelvic cavity signals a condition known as _____.
4. One of the most common symptoms of pregnancy is _____ _____, which may last up to 12 weeks.
5. Diminished gastric motility during pregnancy can cause _____.

6. Flatulence during pregnancy may be due to gas-forming _____ in the intestine.

7. Pressure exerted by the pregnant uterus on the intestines can cause _____.

8. Interference with circulation in the veins during pregnancy can lead to _____ and _____.

9. The pressure of the enlarging uterus on the diaphragm causes _____ _____, which will resolve when _____ occurs.

10. Many pregnant women experience backaches, wearing _____ shoes and practicing good _____ will help minimize this.

11. Leg cramps can also occur. _____ and frequent rest _____ with the feet _____ help relieve this problem.

12. In the hot weather, _____ of the feet may occur.

13. High-risk pregnancies can cause low _____ _____ and premature or brain-damaged _____.

14. Down syndrome generally occurs in women over the age of _____.

15. Prenatal tests including _____, amniocentesis, and blood tests are available to high-risk mothers.

16. Adolescent mothers do not always seek prenatal care because of _____, denial, or lack of _____.

17. A very serious complication that can occur during pregnancy when the mother drinks excessively is known as _____ _____ _____.

18. Examples of high-risk mothers include women who have had a history of spontaneous _____, _____ _____, or difficult pregnancies in the past.

19. Possible signs of miscarriage include _____ associated with abdominal _____ and severe abdominal _____ and bleeding.

20. Danger signals include persistent _____, chills and _____, sudden escape of _____ from the vaginal area, swelling of the face or fingers, and severe headache. If the home health aide notices these signals, the aide needs to _____ _____ _____ _____ _____.

21. Home health aide care for the pregnant woman generally is necessary only if the mother is _____ _____.

22. Five things the home health aide needs to remember when caring for a pregnant client are:

    a. _____

    b. _____

    c. _____

    d. _____

    e. _____

23. Lochia is the bloody vaginal discharge following the normal _____.

24. Lochia should not have a foul _____.

25. Breast _____ is painful. The aide can offer _____ _____ and suggest that the client wear a _____ _____.

26. The perineal incision made during delivery is called an _____.

27. Pain from incisions can be helped by the use of a _____ _____.

28. As the uterus contracts during the postpartum period, the client will have _____. This can be relieved by medication prescribed by the health care provider.

29. The new mother may experience difficulty in _____ for only a short time.

30. A normal fetus will grow in the woman's uterus for approximately _____ days.

True or False. *Answer the following statements true (T) or false (F).*

31. T F Deficiencies in the diet of the mother can result in low birth weight babies.

32. T F Tobacco use during pregnancy generally does not harm the baby.

33. T F Drug-addicted babies can result from drug-addicted mothers.

34. T F Fetal alcohol syndrome causes babies to be underweight and mentally deficient.

35. T F The postpartum period is defined as that period preceding the birth of the child.

36. T F Breast engorgement occurs immediately after delivery.

37. T F The new mother may find that she is sweating more than usual. This is normal.

38. T F Postpartum blues are relatively rare.

39. T F The new mother needs to rest as much as she can.

40. T F Breast-feeding mothers do not need to continue iron and prenatal vitamins.

Multiple Choice. *Choose the correct answer or answers.*

41. Discomforts of pregnancy include
    a. nausea, constipation, heartburn
    b. coughing, temperature
    c. loose stools, high temperature
    d. chest pain, difficulty breathing

42. New mothers are released from hospitals after
    a. 1 week
    b. 3 days
    c. 24 to 48 hours
    d. after 6 days

43. The home health aide caring for a new mother at home should watch for and report to the case manager immediately if the client
    a. is weeping and feeling blue
    b. has bright red vaginal bleeding
    c. has headache and tiredness
    d. all of these

44. Medical factors placing women in high-risk groups include
    a. history of spontaneous abortions, stillbirths, or premature births
    b. women who have cardiac, respiratory, diabetic, hypertensive, or renal disease
    c. have been pregnant five times or more
    d. all of the above

45. Women are often aware of the danger signals of heavy vaginal bleeding, ongoing light spotting, or severe abdominal cramps, which may indicate signs of miscarriage. Other signs include
    a. persistent vomiting
    b. swelling of face or fingers
    c. severe and continuous headache and blurred vision
    d. all of the above

46. Home health aide services for a pregnant mother can occur if
    a. pregnancy is high-risk
    b. mother is under unusual stress
    c. mother is on complete bed rest
    d. none of the above

47. Signs of hypertensive disorders of pregnancy include all but
    a. severe heartburn
    b. elevated blood pressure
    c. protein in the urine
    d. swelling in hands and feet on rising in the morning

48. The home health aide should do all but
    a. watch for vaginal bleeding and signs of infection
    b. provide all care for the infant excluding parents from participation
    c. be aware that emotional changes may range from depression to elation in both parents
    d. help with home management activities

Documentation Exercises. *Read the following descriptions and provide documentation for each scenario.*

49. You are caring for a new mother, Mrs. Pal. She has three other children under the age of 5. You are to care for the family as well as the new mother. The younger children are constantly wanting to bother their mother. What can you do to let Mrs. Pal get some well-deserved rest? Document your response and care provided.

50. You are caring for a client who has recently had a cesarean delivery. She complains of pain in the area of her stitches when she stands. She admits to not performing peri care. What should you do? Document your conversation and care provided.

PRACTICE SITUATIONS

Case 1

Your client is five months pregnant. She is bleeding vaginally. This is her first pregnancy. She is emotionally distraught. You will need to care for her personal care needs and care for her household while she is on bed rest. You know that she is very upset.

Questions

1. What can you do to help her cope with this problem?
2. What activities can she enjoy in bed?
3. Can you think of activities that you can participate in with her?

Case 2

Your client has had a healthy baby girl. You have been hired to help her for a week so that she can get some extra rest before assuming the responsibilities of the entire household. The problem is her friends, who continually pop in to say hi. Your client does not want to tell them to leave.

Questions

1. What can you do to help your client get her needed rest and not insult her friends?
2. Can you work out visiting times with her friends?

CROSSWORD PUZZLE

Across

5 stomach contents backing up into esophagus

9 complication from drinking alcohol during pregnancy

Down

1 feeling of gassiness

2 women placed in high-risk group due to medical conditions

3 period after delivering infant

4 uterus drops into pelvic cavity

6 vaginal discharge after delivery

7 period of depression after delivery

8 rectal varicose veins

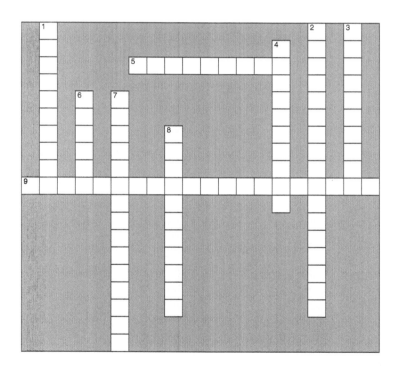

UNIT QUIZ

Short Answer/Fill in the Blanks. *Complete the following sentences with the correct word or words.*

1. _____ is regarded as a normal and natural stage of a woman's life cycle.

2. Extra demands are placed on the woman's body by her growing _____.

3. Four common pregnancy discomforts are frequent _____, morning _____, heartburn or flatulence, and constipation or _____.

4. An _____ test is done usually in the fourth month of pregnancy to check the growth of the fetus.

5. Care of the woman and fetus before childbirth is called _____ _____.

6. List five discomforts of pregnancy.

   a. _____

   b. _____

   c. _____

   d. _____

   e. _____

7. Varicose veins can develop during pregnancy caused by pressure on the great veins of the _____, hereditary predisposition, constrictive clothing, and prolonged _____. Woman should be encouraged to _____ her legs often and wear elastic _____ _____.

8. _____ is a common complaint of pregnant women resulting from adjustments in posture caused by carrying the baby's weight.

9. Complications of pregnancy can affect the health of the _____ and _____. It is important that women receive _____ _____ throughout the pregnancy.

10. The best treatment for leg cramps is _____ the muscles.

True or False. *Answer the following statements true (T) or false (F).*

11. T F   The home health aide should encourage the expectant mother to drink plenty of fluids.

12. T F   Exhaustion is a normal postpartum discomfort.

13. T F   Breast engorgement only occurs in breast-feeding women.

14. T F   Alcohol used in moderation during pregnancy does not affect the fetus.

15. T F   Pregnant women need to take multivitamins with folic acid to prevent birth defects.

16. T F   It is normal for women to have a pale yellow, thin vaginal discharge during pregnancy.

17. T F   Women over age 35 are more likely to give birth to babies with Down syndrome, a form of mental retardation.

18. T F Tobacco use is one of the leading causes of prenatal problems such as vaginal bleeding, miscarriage, and early delivery.

19. T F The reason for frequent blood pressure checks and urine testing for sugar and protein is to determine sex of the child.

20. T F Signs of hypertensive disorder of pregnancy include swelling of feet and ankles.

Matching. *Match each term with the correct definition.*

21. ____ breast engorgement

22. ____ engagement

23. ____ hemorrhoids

24. ____ lochia

25. ____ varicose veins

a. bloody vaginal discharge seen postpartum

b. swollen veins

c. breast milk coming in a few days postdelivery

d. uterus drops into the pelvic cavity

e. enlarged varicose veins around the anus

Multiple Choice. *Choose the correct answer or answers.*

26. A sign of pregnancy is
    a. frequent urination
    b. morning sickness
    c. heartburn
    d. all of these

27. Danger signals in pregnancy may include
    a. persistent vomiting
    b. chills and fever
    c. swelling of face or fingers
    d. all of these

28. Prenatal tests that can determine the health of the fetus include
    a. ultrasound
    b. amniocentesis
    c. blood tests
    d. all of the above

29. Possible signs of miscarriage include all but
    a. varicose veins
    b. bleeding associated with abdominal cramping
    c. heavy vaginal bleeding or light spotting that continues for several days
    d. passing clots or grayish pink material

30. Fetal alcohol syndrome (FAS)
    a. results from drinking alcohol during pregnancy
    b. produces infants who are born underweight
    c. causes mental deficiencies and multiple deformities
    d. all of the above

31. Women are placed in high-risk groups because of medical factors such as
    a. history of spontaneous abortions, stillbirths, or premature births
    b. women who have cardiac, respiratory, diabetic, hypertensive, or renal disease
    c. have been pregnant five times or more
    d. all of the above

32. Signs of hypertensive disorder of pregnancy include
    a. swelling in hands and feet on rising in the morning
    b. elevated blood pressure
    c. protein in the urine
    d. development of hemorrhoids

33. Postpartum discomforts include all but
    a. incisional pain
    b. lochia
    c. heartburn
    d. breast engorgement

34. Home health aide considerations for the postpartum new mother are
    a. Encourage the new mother to get as much rest as possible to regain energy.
    b. Emotional changes may range from depression to elation in both parents: be understanding and patient.
    c. Involve the family in care of the new baby to help the family in adjustment.
    d. Watch for signs of infection and report them to the nurse.
    e. All of the above.

35. Breast-feeding mothers need to
    a. consume 500 to 800 additional calories per day
    b. eat three meals and a bedtime snack at regular intervals
    c. add protein such as meat, eggs, milk, and cheese to diet
    d. calcium, iron, and vitamin supplements should continue
    e. all of the above

UNIT 25   INFANT CARE

LEARNING OBJECTIVES

After studying this unit, you should be able to:
- Describe the different ways a mother may breast-feed her infant
- Explain the steps involved in bottle-feeding an infant
- Describe three techniques for burping an infant
- Describe the steps to bathe an infant
- Define circumcision and identify the appropriate care for the circumcised/ uncircumcised penis
- Explain how to care for the infant's umbilical cord
- Identify safety precautions to be taken with each infant care procedure
- Demonstrate the following:
  Procedure 74   Assisting with Breast-Feeding and Breast Care
  Procedure 75   Bottle-Feeding an Infant
  Procedure 76   Burping an Infant
  Procedure 77   Bathing an Infant

TERMS TO DEFINE

- bottle-feeding
- breast-feeding
- circumcision
- foreskin
- glans
- lactose
- meconium

APPLICATION EXERCISES

Short Answer/Fill in the Blanks. *Complete the following sentences with the correct word or words.*

1. The birth of a baby is an _____ for both parents and the baby.

2. The individuals who meet the infant's primary needs influence his or her _____ and _____ _____.

3. Feeding the infant should be an _____, _____ time.

4. Breast milk is the _____ food for any infant.

5. Bottle-feeding allows members of the family to _____ in feeding the infant.

6. The infant should be placed on his or her abdomen only if _____,
_____ _____ _____, or _____
_____.

7. The infant should be burped after drinking _____ to _____
ounces of formula or between breasts.

8. If the infant is circumcised, the penis should be _____ and covered with
_____ each time the diaper is changed.

9. The redness and the secretions from the circumcision should disappear within
_____ _____.

10. The uncircumcised infant's penis should be cleansed with _____ and
_____.

True or False. *Answer the following statements true (T) or false (F).*

11. T   F   Physical and emotional well-being are intimately related to each other.

12. T   F   Caring for a newborn infant comes naturally to new parents.

13. T   F   Newborn infants will triple their birth weight in one year.

14. T   F   The infant should be placed on his or her abdomen after eating.

15. T   F   After feeding, immediately place infant down for a nap.

Multiple Choice. *Choose the correct answer or answers.*

16. The home health aide's responsibilities for infant care include

  a. assisting with feeding the infant

  b. diaper changes and bathing the infant

  c. noting and reporting to the nurse or case manager any infant feeding, hygiene, or family
  bonding concerns

  d. all of the above

17. When bottle-feeding an infant, you need to

  a. prop the bottle

  b. burp the infant after every 2 to 3 ounces of fluid

  c. place the infant on the stomach after feeding is completed

  d. none of these

18. It is necessary to burp the infant to

  a. prevent the infant from overeating

  b. give the infant a rest from eating

  c. allow removal of air the infant swallowed while eating

  d. all of these

19. Breast milk is the best milk for the infant because

  a. The major ingredients are suited to the infant's needs.

  b. The milk will not be spoiled.

  c. The mother will cuddle the baby while feeding.

  d. All of these.

20. The infant should be given a sponge bath
    a. until the stump of the umbilical cord falls off
    b. to conserve water
    c. twice a day
    d. none of these

21. When the home health aide is bathing the infant, the aide should
    a. notice the skin condition
    b. make sure all the soap is rinsed off the infant
    c. relax and talk softly to the infant
    d. all of these

22. All of the following are important aspects of umbilical cord care except
    a. Keep the cord area dry at all times.
    b. After bathing the infant, wipe the cord area with alcohol.
    c. Keep the diaper folded below the cord area until the cord falls off.
    d. Tape a quarter over the cord area to prevent a hernia.

23. Infants need to be bathed
    a. every day
    b. every two to three days
    c. two times a day
    d. once a week

24. How often should the diaper be changed?
    a. whenever found soiled
    b. every two to three hours after feeding
    c. four times a day
    d. only after bowel movement, due to disposable diaper superabsorbency

25. To prevent urine burns and infection, when changing the diaper
    a. Use toilet paper to remove any stool, then wash perineal area and buttocks using washcloth with mild soap and water or disposable wipes.
    b. Wipe front to back only in females.
    c. Apply moisture-barrier ointment such as Vaseline™, A & D ointment, or Balmex.
    d. All of the above.

Documentation Exercises. *Read the following descriptions and provide documentation for each scenario.*

26. You are caring for an infant, Bobby. He is only 3 days old. Every time you feed him, he vomits. His mother says he has been throwing up since he was born. She has tried two different formulas, but he still vomits. What should you do? Document the patient care provided.

27. You are assigned to care for twins, along with their mother who had cesarean surgery. The care plan includes bathing the infants and assisting the mother with bathing. Additional duties are to prepare meals and launder clothes. Document the care provided.

PRACTICE SITUATIONS

Case 1

You are caring for a client with a 6-week-old infant. You have been hired because the mother is at her wits end. The infant cries constantly. Mrs. Lopes cannot get any rest. She is emotionally unable to cope with the infant. She is convinced that the infant hates her.

Questions

1. What can you do to help the infant?

2. How can you comfort Mrs. Lopes?

3. What can you do to help Mrs. Lopes cope with the infant?

Case 2

You are caring for Baby Maggie. Every time you feed her, she vomits. You have tried different formulas with the same result. Her mother is very concerned that you do not know how to feed infants.

Questions

1. What do you think is happening?

2. How will you explain to the mother that something is seriously wrong with the infant?

3. Should you contact your case manager?

CROSSWORD PUZZLE

Across

3 first stools after birth

4 head of penis

5 breast milk sugar

Down

1 breast-feeding an infant

2 removal of foreskin

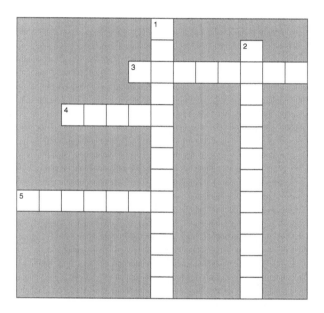

UNIT QUIZ

Short Answer/Fill in the Blanks. *Complete the following sentences with the correct word or words.*

1. During the first year of life, the infant is totally _____ on the care of others.

2. Caring for a newborn can create _____ for new parents.

3. The newborn infant will _____ its birth weight during the first year of life.

4. The two methods of feeding an infant are _____ _____ and _____ _____.

5. _____ _____ is the best possible food for any infant.

6. While breast-feeding, the nursing period is gradually increased from just a few minutes to 20 minutes.

7. To remove the infant's mouth from the breast, have the mother insert _____ in infant's mouth to break the suction.

8. The three positions for breast-feeding are:

   a. _____

   b. _____

   c. _____

9. The first stools the infant will have are called _____ stools.

10. Infant formula combines all the nutrients found in breast milk; however, it does not provide the _____ found in the mother's breast milk.

True or False. *Answer the following statements true (T) or false (F).*

11. T F You should test the temperature of the formula before feeding.

12. T F Breast-fed babies do not need to be burped after feeding.

13. T F The newborn should be given a bath every day.

14. T F You should always check the temperature of the water before placing the infant in the basin.

15. T F When putting the infant down to sleep, place the infant on his or her side or abdomen.

16. T F It is not necessary for the nursing mother to wash the nipple before each feeding, as this can lead to drying and cracking.

17. T F After nursing, it is important to air-dry the nipple.

18. T F The newborn infant will double his or her weight during the first year of life.

19. T F Cracked nipples are common among breast-feeding women.

20. T F Breast milk has infection-fighting properties.

Matching. *Match each term with the correct definition.*

21. _____ circumcision

22. _____ foreskin

23. _____ glans

24. _____ lactose

25. _____ premature

a. infant born before 40 weeks

b. head of penis

c. surgical removal of foreskin

d. skin covering the head of penis

e. sugar in breast milk

Multiple Choice. *Choose the correct answer or answers.*

26. The purpose of assisting with breast-feeding and breast care is

   a. to provide for cleanliness and protect the nipples from cracking or soreness

   b. to protect the infant from infection

   c. to promote mother-infant interaction

   d. all of the above

27. If the infant is getting enough breast milk, the infant should be wetting a diaper how frequently until the infant is 3 months old?

   a. almost hourly

   b. every two to three hours

   c. every four hours

   d. four times a day

28. Bottle-feeding guidelines for the home health aide include all but

   a. Clean all equipment properly, as the newborn infant's immune system is immature.

   b. Correct measurement of formula and water is essential.

   c. Once formula is mixed, it must be refrigerated and used within 72 hours.

   d. Burp the infant after every 2 to 3 ounces.

29. If an infant drinks a partial bottle, you should

   a. cover the nipple for later use

   b. refrigerate covered formula

   c. throw the rest away

   d. add more formula and water to fill the bottle again

30. Care of the umbilical cord involves

   a. When diapering the baby, fold the top of the diaper over so that it does not cover the navel.

   b. Sponge bathe the baby as needed until the cord falls off.

   c. Some health care providers recommend cleaning around the cord stump with a piece of cotton dipped in alcohol.

   d. All of the above.

SECTION 8

Employment

UNIT 26   JOB-SEEKING SKILLS

LEARNING OBJECTIVES

After studying this unit, you should be able to:

- List potential employment sites that hire homemaker/home health aides
- Prepare a personal information sheet
- Describe how to present yourself in a professional manner during an employment interview
- Practice completing an employment application accurately
- Give five examples of misconduct on the job

TERMS TO DEFINE

- information sheet
- infraction
- misconduct
- personal reference
- registry service

APPLICATION EXERCISES

Short Answer/Fill in the Blanks. *Complete the following sentences with the correct word or words.*

1. Your first step toward finding a job is to _____ your community's job market.

2. Three places to look for employment are:

   a. _____

   b. _____

   c. _____

3. When going to the interview, it is better to go _____.

4. You should dress _____ and avoid _____, excessive _____, and _____ for the interview.

5. It is a good idea to arrive at the interview _____.

6. Generally personal references should not include _____.

7. Take care to fill out the application _____ and to follow the instructions exactly.

8. The majority of states have mandatory requirements for hiring _____

_____ _____.

9. Five examples of misconduct on the job are:

a. _____

b. _____

c. _____

d. _____

e. _____

Multiple Choice. *Choose the correct answer or answers.*

10. When the home health aide prepares for the interview, he or she needs to

a. dress neatly

b. have clean, neatly styled hair

c. make eye contact with the interviewer

d. all of these

11. It is important to find out information about a job before accepting it. Some of the information the home health aide needs to consider is

a. the travel distance required

b. the benefits, including insurance and holidays

c. the number of hours of work required

d. all of these

12. Sample appropriate interview questions include all but

a. How many children do you have?

b. Have you had previous homemaker/home health aide work experience?

c. Can you tell me about your previous employment?

d. Why did you leave your last job?

13. To start off the interview

a. Introduce yourself to the interviewer by name with a smile, firm handshake, and make eye contact.

b. Answer all questions truthfully and with more than one word.

c. Only speak positively about former employers and working conditions.

d. All of the above.

14. All of the following need to be brought to the interview except

a. certificate of completion of programs: CPR, First Aid, Home Health Aide training, state certificate

b. skills checklist

c. driver's license and Social Security card

d. homeowner's/renter's insurance

Documentation Exercises. *Read the following descriptions and provide documentation for each scenario.*

15. You accept employment with a home health care agency. When you arrive at the home to be oriented, the case manager tells you that you will be responsible for a 2-week-old infant. You specified on your employment application that you did not feel comfortable caring for newborns. They are counting on you to care for the mother and the infant. How will you handle this situation?

16. You have misplaced your Social Security card. You are scheduled for an appointment to be interviewed in one hour. How will you handle this situation?

17. You have been employed by a home health care agency. You go in to receive your assignment and discover the location of the client is 50 miles from the office. You explained to the interviewer at orientation that you would not be able to travel more than a few miles because your car was not functioning well. The nurse orienting you told you this would not be a problem. What can you do?

18. You arrive 20 minutes early for your job interview. You look for a parking place, but none is available near the location of the agency. Finally, you find a parking place eight blocks from the agency location. You will never make it on time. What could you have done to prevent this situation?

19. Fill out the practice application for employment; refer to Figure 26–1.

CUSHMAN MANAGEMENT ASSOCIATES

APPLICATION FOR EMPLOYMENT

We are an equal opportunity employer. Federal and state laws prohibit discrimination in employment policies based on race, color, religion, sex, age, handicap, disability, or national origin. No question on this application is asked for the purpose of limiting or excluding any applicant's consideration for employment because of his or her race, color, religion, sex, age, handicap, disability, or national origin.

Name: Last First Middle	Social Security No.	Telephone No.

Address: Street City State Zip Code	Licensed Nurses Only	
	Mass. Reg. No.	Date Granted:

If your records may be under a name other than indicated above, please specify:	Last Renewal:	Expiration Date:

Are you a citizen of the United States? ☐ yes ☐ no	If you are not a U.S. Citizen, do you have the legal right to remain permanently in the United States? ☐ yes ☐ no	Explain
Are you between the ages of 18 and 70? ☐ yes ☐ no	Do you know of any fact that would limit or impair your ability to perform the functions of the job you are applying for? ☐ yes ☐ no	Describe

Date of last Physical Examination:	Family Physician:	I authorize my doctor to release to you the results of my pre-employment and subsequent medical examinations, and to discuss those results with you. ☐ yes ☐ no

Position desired:	Hours desired:	Salary expected:

Specialized training or experience not shown on other side of form:

Where now employed?	Reason for desiring change:

Have you ever pleaded guilty or been convicted of a felony? ☐ yes ☐ no   If yes to either, please explain:

or a misdemeanor other than a first conviction for drunkenness, simple assault, speeding, minor traffic violations, affray, or disturbance of the peace within the past 5 years? ☐ yes ☐ no

In case of emergency notify	name relationship
	address telephone

* I authorize the schools, employers, and individuals listed in this application to release any information regarding my previous employment, character, general reputation and personal characteristics.   ☐ yes ☐ no

I certify that the statements I have made in this application are true and hereby grant the employer permission to verify the accuracy and completeness of this information and to investigate all references and educational records. I understand that any false or misleading statements made by me on this application or in conjunction with my physical examination will be sufficient cause for the rejection of this application or for immediate dismissal if such false or misleading information is discovered after my employment. If I am accepted for employment, I agree to abide by the rules and regulations of the employer.

Signed _____

Date _____

"It is unlawful in Massachusetts to require or administer a lie detector test as a condition of employment or continued employment. An employer who violates this law shall be subject to criminal penalties and civil liability."

Figure 26–1

(continues)

TO THE EMPLOYEE

Because you are important to us, we want to help you develop a good work record. If we feel that you are violating any of our rules and policies, or that you have misunderstood the terms of employment, we will hold a conference with you. Continued *infractions* will cause your immediate dismissal. PLEASE READ THE FOLLOWING CAREFULLY.

1. *Attendance and tardiness record:* Recurring cancellations of promised scheduled workdays may result in dismissal. Absence without call in may result in immediate termination. No pay raises will be granted if attendance and tardiness records are unsatisfactory. We must be able to depend on you. You must call in if you are unable to meet your assignment.

2. *Unbecoming conduct:* Any of the following are considered to be gross *misconduct:* carelessness and inattention to client care; failure to perform duties; violation of safe practices; inefficiency and wasting of materials; refusal to obey direct orders; insubordination; rude, discourteous or uncivil behavior; intoxication, drinking, or possession of intoxicating beverages while on duty; gambling on duty; sleeping on duty; unauthorized absence from assignment or leaving early without permission; failure to report an injury or accident concerning an employee or client; soliciting tips from clients or families; sale of services to clients or families; divulging confidential information about client and family; theft and/or dishonesty; *pilferage* of drugs or violation of any law on drug use including use or sale of same; damaging, defacing or mishandling equipment or property; interfering with work performance of another employee; falsifying client or personnel records or any form of misrepresentation.

Employee's statement:

I have read the above rules and regulations and understand my responsibilities to the agency and client. I agree to abide by these terms of employment.

_____   _____
Employee Signature   Date

_____   _____
Supervisor's Signature   Date

Figure 26–1   (continued)

PRACTICE SITUATIONS

Case 1

You have completed your course as a home health aide. You applied for a position as a home health aide with Jones Home Health. You have been asked to come to an interview.

Questions

1. How will you prepare for the interview?

2. What do you need to bring with you?

3. How will you dress for the interview?

Case 2

You have arrived for your 11A.M. interview. You are dressed appropriately. You have your certificates, your driver's license, your health statement, and other various papers. When you are called for your interview, the nurse who is conducting the interview states that you are an hour late. You check your day planner, and sure enough, you were scheduled to be here one hour earlier.

Questions

1. What do you do?

2. How can you let this nurse know that you are very interested in this job?

3. How can you prevent this from happening next time?

CROSSWORD PUZZLE

Across

4 sheet listing facts, usually on job application

5 breaking the rules

Down

1 references from other than family members

2 carelessness and inattention to client care

3 home health aide agency

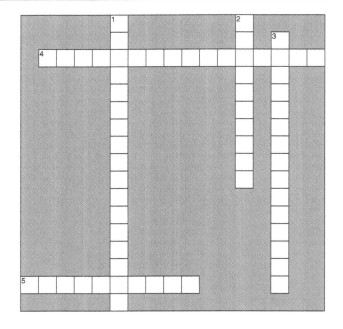

UNIT QUIZ

Short Answer/Fill in the Blanks. *Complete the following sentences with the correct word or words.*

1. Make a _____ of those places you plan to contact; then keep a _____ of the date you called and who you spoke with.

2. The _____ provides you with an opportunity to discuss your skills, but also helps you to learn more about the company, the people you'll work with, company policies, and job details.

3. Arrive at least _____ minutes early for the interview.

4. Have an _____ _____ with you, listing some facts that appear on the application as this will save you time.

5. If you do not have a telephone, you should leave the number of a _____ or friend who has agreed to take messages for you.

6. Read the application form _____ before completing it. Do not leave any items _____; write in "N.A." (not applicable).

7. If you are offered the job, you have the choice of _____ the agency's terms, _____ about it for a few days, or looking elsewhere.

8. The _____ will usually let you know when you will be contacted.

9. To be qualified to operate, agencies now must meet exacting standards set by both the state Department of Health and the _____ for _____ and _____.

True or False. *Answer the following statements true (T) or false (F).*

10. T   F   You should dress neatly for a job interview.

11. T   F   It is acceptable to wear neat shorts and a halter top to an interview.

12. T   F   You should wear excessive jewelry and makeup to an interview.

13. T   F   After an interview, you should send a thank-you letter.

14. T   F   Personal references may be relatives.

Multiple Choice. *Choose the correct answer or answers.*

15. Collect and bring the following items to the interview
    a. résumé, personal references, and record of immunizations
    b. program certificates: home health aide training, CPR, First Aid
    c. driver's license, automobile insurance, and Social Security card
    d. all of the above

16. Before you go to a job interview
    a. Research all you can about the agency.
    b. Plan a travel route to the agency.
    c. Review interview questions and plan how you will answer them.
    d. Practice answering interview questions.
    e. All of the above.

17. Standards for home health agencies include
    a. a grievance procedure for an agency's employees
    b. client's bill of rights that must be explained to the client in the presence of a witness
    c. documentation of certification of all employees
    d. proof of attendance at a minimum number of in-services yearly
    e. all of the above

18. An applicant for a home health aide position must
    a. have proof of citizenship or alien registration
    b. satisfactory completion of a home health aide course
    c. proof of being on the state registry for home health aides
    d. no legal record for client abuse or misuse of client's property

Made in the USA
Lexington, KY
08 December 2012